REVIEW OF

D1490438

ESSENTIAL
PHARMACOLOGY

WITH NURSING IMPLICATIONS
AND SELF-ASSESSMENT QUESTIONS

Katherine Stefos, Ph.D., R.Ph.

M.D. Anderson Hospital and Tumor Institute;
Consultant, University of Texas Health Science
Center—Houston, School of Nursing, Houston, Texas

APPLETON & LANGE
Norwalk, Connecticut/San Mateo, California

0-8385-8417-9

Notice: Our knowledge in clinical sciences is constantly changing. As new information becomes available, changes in treatment and in the use of drugs become necessary. The author(s) and the publisher of this volume have taken care to make certain that the doses of drugs and schedules of treatment are correct and compatible with the standards generally accepted at the time of publication. The reader is advised to consult carefully the instruction and information material included in the package insert of each drug or therapeutic agent before administration. This advice is especially important when using new or infrequently used drugs.

Copyright © 1988 by Appleton & Lange
A Publishing Division of Prentice Hall

All rights reserved. This book, or any parts thereof, may not be used or reproduced in any manner without written permission. For information, address Appleton & Lange, 25 Van Zant Street, East Norwalk, Connecticut 06855.

88 89 90 91 92 / 10 9 8 7 6 5 4 3 2 1

Prentice-Hall International (UK) Limited, *London*
Prentice-Hall of Australia Pty. Limited, *Sydney*
Prentice-Hall Canada, Inc., *Toronto*
Prentice-Hall Hispanoamericana, S.A., *Mexico*
Prentice-Hall of India Private Limited, *New Delhi*
Prentice-Hall of Japan, Inc., *Tokyo*
Simon & Schuster Asia Pte. Ltd., *Singapore*
Editora Prentice-Hall do Brasil Ltda., *Rio de Janeiro*
Prentice-Hall, *Englewood Cliffs, New Jersey*

Library of Congress Cataloging-in-Publications Data

Stefos, Katherine.
    Review of essential pharmacology : with nursing implications and self-assessment questions / Katherine Stefos.
        p. cm.
    Bibliography: p.
    ISBN 0-8385-8417-9
    1. Pharmacology—Handbooks, manuals, etc. 2. Nursing—Handbooks, manuals, etc. I. Title.
    [DNLM: 1. Drug Therapy—examination questions. 2. Drug Therapy—nurses' instruction. 3. Pharmacology—examination questions.
    4. Pharmacology—nurses' instruction. QV 4 S8175r]
    RM301.12.S74 1988
    615'.1—dc19
    DNLM/DLC   88-3467
    for Library of Congress   CIP

Acquisitions Editor: Marion K. Welch
Production Editor: Charles F. Evans
Designer: Kathleen Peters Ceconi

PRINTED IN THE UNITED STATES OF AMERICA

To all the dedicated nurses
especially
Karen, Donna, Mary, Sue, and Jan

Contents

Preface

The principles of pharmacology are often regarded as one of the more difficult areas of study. The difficulty, however, does not lie in the material content per se, but rather in the great body of knowledge that exists and the continuous addition of new advances in drug therapy. With this in mind, this book was designed to give nursing students, graduates, and others in allied health-related sciences a basic review. The organizational format of the book was developed in order to help these individuals formulate their own unique means of assimilating the extensive amount of material needed to be competent and knowledgeable in this area.

Representative drug classes have been selected for presentation to demonstrate various pharmacological principles and to give a broad overview of the area. All chapters follow a similar format. Each one begins with an introduction providing the reader with an orientation to a particular drug class. This is followed by drug action and fate, uses, side and adverse effects, contraindications and cautions, and nursing implications. Other pertinent information may be given in some of the chapters when considered necessary to enhance the understanding of that drug class. A table summarizing representative drugs is included in each chapter. Drugs are listed by generic name with trade names and other applicable information. At the end of each chapter is a list of questions that allows the reader to review and assess his or her understanding of that chapter.

This book may be used in conjunction with a textbook in a formal academic class. In addition, it can be used as a review for nursing state board examinations, as a guide in nursing and related personnel orientation programs in health care facilities, and by individuals in other health-related sciences desiring a broad review of pharmacology.

K.S.
Houston, Texas

Reviewers

Cathy Bevil, Ed.D., R.N.
College of New Rochelle
New Rochelle, New York

Virginia Britton, R.N.

Rosemarie Hogan, R.N., M.S.N.
Kent State University
Kent, Ohio

Diane Lapkin, Ed.D., R.N.
Middlesex County College
Bedford, Massachusetts

Elizabeth Pennington, Ed.D.
University of Michigan
Ann Arbor, Michigan

Acknowledgments

In the preparation of this book, certain events and individuals influenced its progress in various ways. I want to thank Marion Kalstein-Welch of Appleton & Lange for her encouragement during the initial stages of this project. Many thanks go to Joan Fox for her expert deciphering of my handwriting and her typing abilities and to Denise Stracener for her assistance throughout the preparation of the manuscript, especially the nursing implications, and for her gentle nudging to complete this project. Lastly, I would like to recognize all the students in my classes through the years without whom this project would not have been conceived.

K.S.
Houston, Texas

1

Review of General Principles and Nursing Implications

Pharmacology is defined as the study of drugs including their chemical properties, actions, and uses. It is without a doubt one of the most dynamic fields of study, rapidly changing, with new drugs and new drug classes constantly being developed. At times, it seems practically impossible to keep abreast of all the new developments; however, it is of utmost importance for all health professionals to stay informed in order to provide adequate care to patients. More specifically, current knowledge pertaining to drugs is especially important to the nurse. The nurse occupies a unique position on the health team related to drug therapy. The physician's role is to diagnose and prescribe appropriate therapy, the pharmacist reviews the order and dispenses, and the nurse administers the medication. Being the last individual in this chain of events does not lessen the responsibility of the nurse. In fact, the nurse is the last "check point" prior to the medication entering the patient's body. In addition, the nurse is in the best position to observe the effects of the medication. It is important to note and communicate not only the desired effects but also the undesirable effects, i.e., the side and adverse effects.

It is the goal of this introductory unit to orient the reader to general principles of pharmacology, major aspects of drug administration, general nursing implications of drug administration, and pharmacological terminology. This unit should serve as preparation to better understand the information presented in the subsequent units.

PHARMACOKINETICS

The pharmacokinetics of a drug is the study of how it is absorbed into the body and at what rate, how long it takes to reach its site of action, and how long and in what manner it is finally eliminated from the body. The pharmacokinetics of a drug, therefore, involve its absorption, distribution, metabolism (or biotransformation), and eventual elimination from the body.

Figure 1–1 is a general schematic representation of what happens to a drug after it is absorbed and enters the circulatory system. Notice that as the drug is circulating in the blood it may complex (attach to) plasma proteins, in which case that portion of the drug is pharmacologically inactive. Another portion of the drug may enter tissue storage sites such as adipose tissue, in which case this portion of the drug is also considered to be inactive. Only the circulating free drug is able to exert a pharmacological effect or effects. The implications of the portion of the drug that is complexed to plasma proteins or stored in adipose

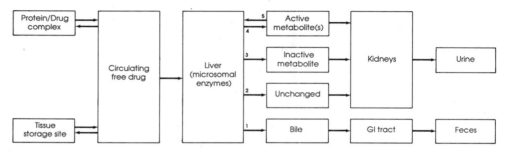

Figure 1–1. Once drugs enter the circulatory system they all circulate through the liver. However, not all drugs are changed or metabolized prior to excretion. Some drugs are concentrated in the liver and excreted via the bile (pathway 1). A drug that falls into this category is the antibiotic erythromycin. Some drugs like the penicillins and cephalosporins are excreted unchanged as active drug (pathway 2). Other drugs are metabolized to inactive products or metabolites before they can be excreted (pathway 3). Morphine is eliminated from the body in this manner. Drugs may be excreted from the body via the kidneys in two other ways: 1. as active metabolites (pathway 4), or 2. as several metabolites, some of which may be excreted as is, others requiring further metabolism prior to elimination (pathways 4 and 5). An example drug in the first instance is the antidiabetic agent chlorpropamide; an example drug in the second instance is the antianxiety agent diazepam.

tissue are that it will be more slowly eliminated from the body. This portion of the drug (in both cases) will become free drug only as the concentration of the circulating free drug decreases. Drugs, for example, with a high percent of plasma protein binding can have a prolonged effect on the individual even after it has been discontinued.

Circulating free drug will pass through the liver, the major organ involved in detoxification. Located in the liver is a group of enzymes collectively known as the microsomal enzymes. These enzymes are responsible for ultimately changing drug molecules into a form that can be easily eliminated from the body. There are exceptions to this process and some drugs are excreted unchanged. Figure 1–1 lists examples of drugs that are exceptions. Others may be changed to another form of the drug that has the same pharmacological effect as the parent drug. These molecules are known as active metabolites. Some drugs and their metabolites require more than one exposure to the liver enzymes to be finally changed into products that can be eliminated from the body.

What are the implications of knowing how a drug is eliminated? Drugs that must be metabolized in the liver prior to elimination are given with close monitoring and at lower doses in those patients with liver disease or with decreased liver function (the elderly or neonates). Drugs that are excreted with no metabolic change via the kidneys, the major organ of elimination, must be given with close monitoring and at lower doses and/or at less frequent intervals in those with decreased kidney function. A minor elimination pathway for some drugs is a concentrating of the drug in the liver and its subsequent elimination in the feces via the bile.

The first step in the action of a drug in the body is its absorption. The drug must enter the circulatory system in order to reach its site of action. How easily, how fast, and to what extent the drug will be systematically absorbed depends on the chemical properties of the drug itself, the route of administration, and dosage form.

For the drug to be absorbed it must be sufficiently lipid soluble to pass through the various membrane barriers and sufficiently water soluble to dissolve in the blood. This means the drug must exist in two states if this is to be accomplished: a charged or ionized state, which is water soluble, and a noncharged or nonionized state, which is lipid soluble (Figs. 1–2 and 1–3). This indeed is the

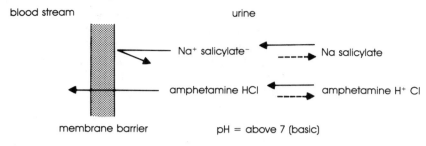

Figure 1–2. In a basic pH, a drug that is a weak acid will predominately be in the ionized or water-soluble form and will not readily penetrate the membrane barrier. The example shown here is sodium salicylate. The opposite is true though for a drug that is a weak base. Notice that the nonionized form will predominate and more of this drug will phetamine. (*Adapted from Meyers FH, Jawetz E, Goldfien A [eds]: Review of Medical Pharmacology, ed 7, Los Altos, Calif, Lange Medical Publications, 1980, with permission.*)

case with most drugs since most are either a weak acid or a base. This means that when in solution some of the drug molecules are ionized and some are not.

The other parameter mentioned that influences the absorption of a drug was route of administration. The slowest absorption occurs when drugs are given orally. There are many membranes that must be transversed; in addition, stomach acidity can destroy a percentage of the drug or the drug can complex with food particles and not be absorbed. Another point for consideration is that drugs absorbed from the gastrointestinal tract enter the circulatory system via the hepatic portal system. This means the drug will initially pass through the liver. For most drugs this is not a problem, but for some this first pass will totally metabolize and render them inactive. These latter drugs are described as being susceptible to the "first pass effect" and are not usually given orally. The way to bypass the liver totally is to administer the drug directly into the circulatory system. Routes that achieve this are the intravenous (IV), sublingual (SL), buccal, and rectal routes. The intramuscular (IM) route will bypass the liver to some extent but not as completely as the routes mentioned.

The other factor that influences the rate of drug absorption is its dosage form. The smaller the particle size, the more completely the drug is dissolved in a solution, the more quickly it will be absorbed. Therefore, a drug solution is more quickly and more completely absorbed than a suspension. A medication formulated as a powder in a capsule is more quickly and more completely absorbed than a medication contained in a compressed tablet.

In some cases rapid absorption is not desired. In this case, long-acting or sustained-action dosage forms are formulated. Slow release medications given

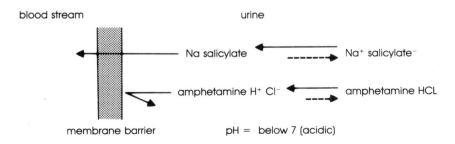

Figure 1–3. The opposite condition is shown in this figure. The pH of the urine is acidic and as might be expected the drug that is the weak acid readily penetrates the membrane barrier because its nonionized form predominates in an acid pH. The opposite is true at this pH for a drug that is a weak base. (*Adapted from Meyers FH, Jawetz E, Goldfien A [eds]: Review of Medical Pharmacology, ed 7, Los Altos, Calif, Lange Medical Publications, 1980, with permission.*)

orally are given for two purposes, either to provide relief for an extended period of time as is the case for antihistaminic products or to delay the release of a substance that may be irritating to the stomach. Another type of formulation delays the release of the medication until the tablet has reached the small intestines. These tablets are enteric coated, which means the outer coating on the tablet will not dissolve until it reaches a site in the gastrointestinal tract that has a basic pH and this is in the small intestines. Medications so formulated are those that are highly irritating to the stomach lining or those that are destroyed by the acid pH in the stomach.

Injectables can also be formulated for sustained absorption. These preparations are *never* given intravenously. They may be given intramuscularly or subcutaneously. Not only is particle size involved, but also the substance or solution in which the drug is dissolved. Penicillin G is formulated into a very thick suspension with benzothine or procaine. This is called a repository preparation and permits the injection of one large dose, which will be absorbed slowly over 2 to 3 days. The same principle is applied to male and female hormones. These drugs are dissolved in oil and one injection may last up to 3 weeks. Another example of sustained release injection are the various insulin preparations other than regular insulin.

Another parameter applicable to the kinetics of a drug is the drug's half-life ($t_{1/2}$). This parameter is defined as the time it takes for half the concentration of the drug to be cleared from the bloodstream. For some drugs, the half-life may be minutes (30 minutes for penicillin G) or it may be in hours (36 hours for digoxin). The half-life of a drug is used in two ways. Drugs with a short half-life should be dosed more frequently than drugs with a long half-life. Compare the dosing interval of every 4 to 6 hours for penicillin G to a once-daily dosing for digoxin. Also multiplying the half-life of a drug by 5 will give the length of time it will take to reach the therapeutic blood level of a drug with normal dosing, and the length of time the drug is essentially cleared from the bloodstream once it has been discontinued.

PHARMACODYNAMICS

Pharmacodynamics is the study of the actions of drugs on the body. There are several ways drugs exert their effects. The most common way is by interacting with specific receptors. Receptors are components or sites located on cells. Drugs that bind or interact with specific receptors and produce a response are called agonists. Drugs that bind with receptors but block a response are called antagonists. Some drugs possess both actions; in that case they are labeled as an agonist/antagonist.

The receptors with which drugs interact are in reality natural components of cells that can be stimulated by substances normally found in the body. Some receptors that have been identified are those for endorphins (opioid receptors), estrogens, steroids, and neurotransmitters (e.g., norepinephrine, acetylcholine, and dopamine).

To further explain the significance of receptors, the adrenergic portion of the nervous system will be used as a model. The adrenergic system contains four types of receptors: alpha 1, alpha 2, beta 1, and beta 2 receptors. All these receptor types will produce a response when stimulated except the alpha 2 receptors, which have a regulatory function.

The responses produced by stimulating alpha 1, beta 1, and beta 2 receptors are listed in Table 1–1. The primary neurotransmitters in the adrenergic system are epinephrine and norepinephrine. Figure 1–4 shows how by stimulating an adrenergic neuron, the neurotransmitter is released, interacts with the receptor, and then is disposed of either by enzyme destruction or re-uptake into the nerve terminal and re-entry into the storage granule.

TABLE 1–1. ORGAN RESPONSES TO SYMPATHETIC NERVE IMPULSES

Organ	Response to Sympathetic (Adrenergic) Impulses	
	Receptor	*Response*
Cardiovascular System		
Heart		
Sinoatrial node	Beta 1	Increased heart rate
Atrioventricular node	Beta 1	Increased automaticity and conduction velocity
Ventricles	Beta 1	Increased force of contraction and conduction velocity
Arterioles (smooth muscle)		
Coronary	Alpha, beta 2, dopaminergic	Constriction and dilatation
Skin and mucosa	Alpha	Constriction
Skeletal muscle	Cholinergic	Dilatation
Cerebral	Alpha	Slight constriction
Mesenteric	Alpha, beta 2, dopaminergic	Constriction and dilatation
Renal	Alpha, beta 2, dopaminergic	Constriction and dilatation
Veins	Alpha, beta 2	Constriction and dilatation
Lung		
Bronchial muscle	Beta 2	Relaxation (bronchodilatation)
Bronchial glands	—	Inhibition
Gastrointestinal tract		
Motility	Alpha, beta 2	Relaxation (decreased motility)
Sphincters	Alpha	Contraction
Exocrine glands	?	Decreased secretion
Salivary glands	Alpha	Constriction: thick, viscous secretion
Gallbladder and ducts	—	Relaxation
Kidney	Beta 2	Renin secretion
Urinary bladder		
Detrusor muscle	Beta 2	Relaxation
Sphincter	Alpha	Contraction
Eye		
Radial muscle	Alpha	Contraction (mydriasis)
Iris	—	—
Ciliary muscle	—	No innervation
Liver	Beta	Glycogenolysis, gluconeogenesis
Pancreas		
Acini	Alpha	Decreased secretion
Islets (beta cells)	Alpha	Decreased secretion
Skin	Beta 2	Increased secretion
Sweat glands	Cholinergic	Increased sweating
Pilomotor muscle	—	Contraction (gooseflesh)
Lacrimal glands	—	No innervation
Nasopharyngeal glands	—	No innervation
Male sex glands	—	Ejaculation

Knowing the structure of the natural substances that stimulate the various receptors allows pharmacologists to produce synthetic compounds that can either mimic the natural substances and produce a response (agonists) or compounds that interact with receptors but produce no effect, receptor blockers (antagonists). Using the adrenergic system again as our model, there are drugs that are classed as alpha or beta receptor stimulants (sympathomimetic agents) or agents that block these receptors (sympatholytic agents).

To demonstrate how this knowledge has been put to use, let us look specifically at the beta receptors that are primarily located in the heart and lungs. Stimulation of the beta receptors will cause an increase in heart rate and bronchodilatation; blocking these receptors will cause the reverse action in these two

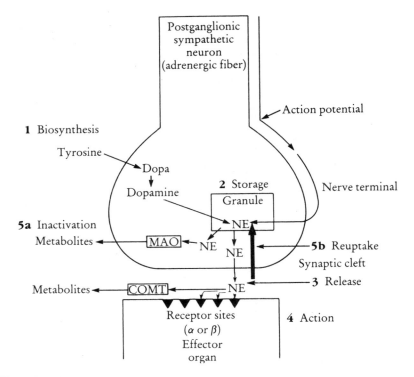

Figure 1–4. Schematic diagram of sympathetic postganglionic neuron showing steps in adrenergic transmission at the neuroeffector junction. 1. *Biosynthesis* of norepinephrine (NE): Tyrosine is taken up by the nerve terminal and converted to dopamine, which after transport into the storage granule is finally synthesized into NE. 2. *Storage:* Following synthesis, NE is stored in the granule until the arrival of a nerve impulse. 3. *Release:* Action potential along the neuron stimulates release of NE from the granule; NE then diffuses into the synaptic cleft to the receptor site of the effector cell. 4. *Action:* The interaction of NE with the receptor sites (α or β) results in a motor response. 5a. *Inactivation of NE:* Enzymatic metabolism of NE occurs within the neuron by action of the enzyme monamine oxidase (MAO) or outside the neuron by the enzyme catechol-O-methyltransferase (COMT). 5b. *Re-uptake* of NE: re-uptake into the nerve terminal and re-entry into the storage granule (*heavy arrow*) comprise another method of removal of NE. (*Reproduced from Hahn AB: Mosby's Pharmacology in Nursing. St. Louis, C.V. Mosby, 1986, with permission.*)

organs. Therefore, in the treatment of asthma, one would use a beta stimulant; for hypertension or angina a beta blocker is used. However, if the individual has asthma in the latter case, treatment with a beta blocker may precipitate an asthma attack. Luckily, subtle differences have been found between heart beta receptors (beta 1 receptors) and those found in the lungs (beta 2 receptors). The goal therefore is to design drugs that would react more specifically with a particular receptor subtype. Many cardiovascular drugs have been developed based on receptor stimulation or blockade.

It is also important to mention other basic ways drugs act to produce their effects. One is as replacement, that is, the substance that is not being synthesized in the body is administered, as in the case of insulin administration in diabetes mellitus. Another means of drug action is the interference or inhibition of a normal biochemical or biologic process. For example, penicillins inhibit the action of an enzyme needed in the synthesis of the bacteria cell wall. The antigout medication allopurinol inhibits the enzyme that converts hypoxanthine to uric acid. Some drugs may interfere with normal physiological processes. It is thought that tricyclic antidepressants elevate the concentration of norepinephrine and serotonin in the neural synapse by blocking the re-uptake pump (see step 5b in Figure 1–4). Some drugs may exert their action by altering cell membrane permeability. This action is exerted by several of the antifungal agents.

GENERAL ASPECTS OF NURSING IMPLICATIONS OF DRUG ADMINISTRATION

This section focuses on the nursing aspects of drug administration and other general information pertaining to drugs.

First, a general review will be given on how drugs are legally classified. Figure 1–5 shows that first, drugs are classed based on whether they require a prescription or not in order to be purchased by the consumer. Those that do not require a prescription are known as over-the-counter (OTC) medications; those that do require a prescription are known as legend drugs. They will have imprinted on their label the following: "Caution: Federal law prohibits dispensing without a prescription." In the hospital, however, regardless of whether a drug is an OTC or legend drug, it cannot be dispensed from the pharmacy without a valid physician's order.

Figure 1–5 also shows that legend drugs are further divided into noncontrolled and controlled substances.

Noncontrolled medications are those drugs used to treat either certain conditions on a short-term basis (e.g., antibiotics) or those drugs used for an indefinite time to manage a chronic condition (e.g., antihypertensives). However, what specifically distinguishes noncontrolled drugs from controlled ones is the potential for psychological and/or physiological addiction of the controlled drugs. Controlled drugs are classed as analgesics, hypnotics, central nervous system stimulants, antianxiety agents, cough suppressants, and antidiarrheal agents.

Controlled drugs are grouped into classes according to their addiction potential. The addiction potential lessens as the class number increases. Therefore, a Class II (CII) drug has more addiction potential than a Class V (CV) drug. Drugs designated as Class I (CI) not only have the most potential for addiction but they also may have hallucinatory properties, and they have no approved

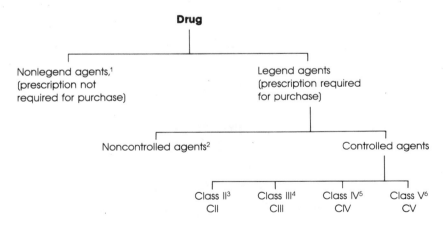

Example drugs and classes of drugs for the designated categories.

1. antihistamines, antacids, exempt CVs such as parepectolin.
2. birth control tablets, antihypertensives
3. morphine, meperidine (Demerol), codeine
4. glutethimide (Doriden)
5. diazepam (Valium), chlordiazepoxide (Librium)
6. diphenoxylate (in Lomotil)

Figure 1–5. Drug categories according to legal requirements.

TABLE 1–2. CLASSES OF CONTROLLED DRUGS

Class	Definition	Comments	Examples
Schedule I (CI)	Drugs and other substances with high potential for abuse or addiction and with no current accepted medical use	Available with special permit to research facilities for investigational use only	marijuana, LSD, peyote
Schedule II (CII)	Drugs with high potential for abuse and addiction with current accepted medical use	Outpatient prescription valid for 2 days only with no refills and written for an amount adequate for 1 month's supply. Inpatient orders valid for 72 hours after which a new order must be written	opium, cocaine, amphetamines, morphine
Schedule III (CIII)	Drugs with less potential for abuse and addiction with current accepted medical use	Outpatient prescription valid for 6 months and may have 5 refills; quantity should not exceed 1 month's supply. Inpatient order usually valid for 7 days	glutethimide, codeine with acetaminophen or aspirin
Schedule IV (CIV)	Drugs with a low potential for addiction and abuse with current accepted medical indication of use	Same as CIIIs	Long-acting barbiturates, depressants, benzotracts
Schedule V (CV)	Drugs with a very low potential for abuse and addiction with current accepted medical indication of use	Same as CIIIs	Lomotil, mixtures that contain limited quantities of opioids

indication for use. This is not to say that Class I drugs are never encountered in a clinical setting. Some may be used investigationally in studies to evaluate their potential effectiveness. This was the case when tetrahydrocannabinols (THC), the active component in marijuana, was evaluated for its antinausea properties prior to its approval. See Table 1–2 for the definitions of the various classes of controlled drugs.

MEDICATION ORDERS

Valid Orders

All medications given to individuals as inpatients are administered per a medication order written by a physician. A valid order is one that contains the following essential information: patient name, hospital number, room number, date, medication name, dose, route, dosing interval, and physician's signature. As needed (PRN) orders should also include the purpose of the medication. The order should be clearly written, leave no room for doubt, and be appropriate for the patient. If there is any aspect of the order that is questionable, it must be clarified with the physician. There are certain other considerations for specific medications that must be addressed. For example, in most hospitals, valid orders for antibiotics must be written on an antibiotic order form. These forms not only include the antibiotics ordered but also document the organism present.

Another consideration when evaluating the validity of an order is whether or not the medication ordered has an automatic stop time. Drugs that fall into this category are antibiotics and controlled substances. Orders for antibiotics expire in 5 to 7 days (depending on hospital policy), orders for Class II drugs expire in 72 hours, and orders for Classes III, IV, and V drugs in 5 to 7 days. In order to continue giving these medications, a new order must be written by the physician once their expiration date has been reached.

Types of Medication Orders

There are different types of medication orders with which the nurse should be familiar. There are routine orders, one time orders, stat orders, now orders, verbal orders (VO), and telephone orders (TO). The most commonly encountered one is the routine order. Medications ordered in this way are given until the physician discontinues the order or the stop time is reached. A single or one time order is written when a drug is administered once at a specific time, for example, cefamandol 2 Gm IV on call to OR. A stat order is written in an emergency life-threatening situation for a drug that is to be administered immediately. An example of this type of order is: epinephrine 1 : 1000 IV stat for allergic reaction. A now order is written when a medication is to be administered for a serious situation as soon as possible but is not considered to be a medical emergency, for example, Valium 5 mg PO now for anxiety. A verbal order is one given orally by the physician to a licensed nurse. This can occur, for example, during a procedure such as intubation when the physician is involved with patient treatment and is unable to write in the chart at that moment. The order is written in the chart and signed off by the nurse followed by VO and the physician's name. To validate the order, the physician must cosign the order within 24 hours. A telephone order is similar to a verbal order, only it is given over the telephone to a licensed nurse. The same procedure is followed when recording the order in the chart, except the nurse notes it as a TO followed by the physician's name. This order must also be signed by the physician within 24 hours. For a list of commonly used medical abbreviations, see the Appendix.

THE NURSE'S ROLE IN DRUG ADMINISTRATION

The nurse has the most constant and consistent access to the patient in the hospital. She or he serves as the last check in protecting the patient from errors and adverse effects of drug therapy. In addition, the nurse is charged with ensuring that none of the five patient rights related to drug administration are violated (Table 1–3). In order to achieve these goals, the nurse should constantly monitor and assess the patient's responses. Nurses can adequately perform this responsibility if the following are kept in mind: (1) indication of use for the drug; (2) purpose of the drug treatment; (3) expected therapeutic outcome; (4) side and adverse effects; (5) allergic reactions; (6) means of absorption, metabolism, and excretion of the drug; and (7) factors that would alter the therapeutic effectiveness of the drug. Thus, the nurse assesses all parameters indicative of drug effectiveness and side and adverse effects and is prepared to intervene appropriately to enhance the beneficial effect and lessen the detrimental effects.

In addition to ensuring the patient's rights, there are certain essential safety measures that should be observed by the nurse in the actual preparation and administration of drugs in order to avoid medication errors. It is important to

---

TABLE 1–3. THE FIVE "RIGHTS"

The five "rights" of a patient that relate to drug administration are:	1. Right drug
	2. Right dose
	3. Right route
	4. Right time
	5. Right patient

always thoroughly wash hands prior to preparing medications. It is best to work alone concentrating on the task at hand and avoiding distracting conversation. A drug should never be given that is prepared by another nurse. Medications should not be touched both for the patient's and nurse's safety. If medication does accidently contaminate the skin, the area should be thoroughly rinsed with plain water first and then washed with soap. The nurse should ensure that the patient has swallowed the medication(s) before leaving the patient, and never leave the medication in the room with the patient promising to take it later. The medication card should always be filled out before administering a drug. The medication label should be read and compared with the medication card at least three times. The patient's name on the identification band must always be compared to the name on the medication card. As an additional safety measure, the patient can be addressed by both first and last name to ensure positive identification.

After the medication(s) is administered, the nurse records the dose(s) given on the Kardex or Medication Administration Record (MAR). Only those medications the nurse has given personally are recorded. Information recorded includes drug name, dose, route, and time of administration. On a MAR form, this information is preprinted and the nurse initials the doses given. Just as important as recording administered medications is the recording of refused or omitted doses and the reason why the medication was not taken by the patient. Additional notes that are made include the beneficial as well as adverse effects of medications and any patient complaints. Record keeping and notations are made immediately after giving the medication(s), never before or at the end of the shift.

The procedure just described applies to routine medications. For all Class II and designated Class III and IV drugs, additional record keeping is required. In order to understand why the additional record keeping is needed, it is necessary first to describe how controlled drugs are delivered to nursing units. Controlled drugs are supplied to nursing units in a way that differs from noncontrolled drugs. Controlled drugs are delivered to the nursing unit as a stock supply directly from the pharmacy. Hence, these drugs are floor stock and the doses on hand are not designated for any particular patient. Controlled drugs are stored in each nursing unit in a special locked cabinet to be used only when they are ordered for a patient.

When pharmacy personnel deliver floor stock controlled drugs, the number of tablets, capsules, or milliliters of the drug is recorded on a narcotic record sheet that accompanies the delivery. The nurse counts and verifies the count and signs the narcotic record sheet and keeps a copy. The number of doses of the controlled drug delivered is also recorded on the narcotic sign-out sheet that is kept on the unit. At all times, the number of doses recorded on the sign-out sheet must correspond to the number of doses on hand. Therefore, when a controlled substance is administered, the routine records are made and also the number of units used is recorded and subtracted from the stock supply to give the actual total on hand. Any dose or partial dose that is not used and is wasted is so noted and initialed by both the nurse who wasted the dose and one who is the witness. At the change of shift, all floor stock controlled drugs are counted by two nurses, one coming on duty and one going off. The counts are then matched against the recorded number. Any discrepancies are reported on an incident report form. As a further safeguard against diversion, pharmacists conduct audits at regular intervals to verify the completeness of the record-keeping procedure.

Stock replacement of controlled drugs is made by pharmacy personnel on a regular basis. Should a controlled drug be ordered that is not routinely stocked, either the licensed nurse may come to the pharmacy to obtain the drug or pharmacy personnel may deliver it. In either case, the records must be updated to indicate the delivery.

It is important to be familiar with those controlled medications that are floor stock and to be aware that the delivery procedure is not the same as with routine medications. These precautions and the extensive record keeping are required in order to comply with the federal law that requires that an accurate count of all Class II drugs be kept in all pharmacies and health care facilities at all times. There can be other controlled drugs in addition to Class II drugs that are also designated as floor stock. They are thus designated as floor stock at the discretion of the particular hospital. This explains why in some hospitals diazepam (Valium CIV) is floor stock and in others it is not. If a Class III, IV, or V drug is designated as floor stock, the same delivery and recording procedures are followed.

DRUG ERRORS

Any time a medication is administered incorrectly, it is considered to be a drug error. In this case, the head nurse or charge nurse is notified, the patient's vital signs are taken and other pertinent observations are made and noted, and the physician is notified, and any remedial measures ordered by the physician are administered. An incident report form is filled out documenting the entire incident clearly. This includes the error, patient assessment data, the presence or absence of any adverse effects, steps taken, and all parties notified.

ROUTES OF ADMINISTRATION

The major routes of administration are the oral (enteral) route and the routes that bypass the gastrointestinal tract: the parenteral routes. The parenteral routes are most often associated with injections, e.g., IV, IM, SQ (subcutaneous). However, the parenteral route would also include any route other than oral ingestion, such as sublingual, rectal, and inhalation. Both routes of administration have their advantages and disadvantages. See Table 1–4 for a list of routes of administration.

The oral route is by far the easiest, safest, most convenient, and most economical means of giving medications. The disadvantages, however, are slow and erratic systemic absorption of the medication. A variety of factors can influence the absorption of medication from the gastrointestinal tract, such as the presence of food, diarrhea, local irritation, and vomiting. Another factor that delays systemic absorption is the numerous membranes that the drug must penetrate in

TABLE 1–4. MAIN ROUTES OF ADMINISTRATION FOR MEDICATIONS

Route	Comments
Oral	
By mouth (PO)	Medication swallowed and usually absorbed in the small intestine
Sublingual (SL)	Medication placed under the tongue and allowed to dissolve
Buccal	Medication placed between cheek and gum and allowed to dissolve
Parenteral	
Intravenous (IV)	Medication injected directly into the vein either as in infusion piggybacks (IVPB), or IV soluset (IVSS), or IV push (IVP)
Intrasmuscular (IM)	Medication injected into the muscle at 45 to 90 degree angle
Subcutaneous (SQ)	Medication injected under the skin at 15 degree angle
Intradermal (ID)	Medication injected under the dermis layer parallel to skin surface
Rectal	Medication inserted into rectum and absorbed through the mucous membrane
Intrathecal (IT)	Medication injected directly into the cavity of the brain

TABLE 1–5. EXAMPLES OF VARIOUS DOSAGE FORMS AND REPRESENTATIVE EXAMPLES

Form	Example	Comments

Capsule
  Sustained release
  capsule
	ampicillin
	Ornade
		Powdered form of medication enclosed in a gelatin capsule

Elixir	phenobarbital elixir	Clear fluid in which drug is dissolved in alcohol and water and sweetened
Solution	Tinactin solution	Clear fluid in which drug is dissolved in water
Suppository	aspirin	Solid dosage form usually inserted in the rectum or vagina designed to melt at body temperature and releases the medication to be absorbed through the surrounding tissue
Suspension	phenytoin suspension NPH insulin	Fine drug particles suspended in fluid that may be given PO, IM, SQ. Always shake well before use
Syrup	promethazine syrup	Medication dissolved in a concentrated sucrose solution

Tablet
  Slow release
  Enteric coated
  Buccal
  Sublingual
	
	Slow K
	Ecotrin
	methyltestosterone
	nitroglycerin
		Solid dosage form in which the medication is compressed with other inert material. They may be given orally, vaginally, buccally, or sublingually. The slow release tablets are formulated with the drug embedded in a matrix or in layers; this allows for a sustained release of the drug over an extended period of time. Enteric-coated tablets are designed to release the medication at a pH that dissolves the outer coating of the tablet. This is done to either protect the stomach from the medication or to protect the medication from the low pH of the stomach

Tincture	tincture of benzoin	Concentrated alcoholic solution of a drug

Topical
  Transdermal patch
  Paste
	
	scopolamine
	nitroglycerin
		These are recent additions to the dosage forms available. The patches contain the medication and slowly release it systemically through the dermis. The paste is applied topically and is systemically absorbed

Troche	Chloraseptic	Solid dosage forms that are allowed to dissolve in the mouth. The action of the medication is intended for in the mouth or throat

order to reach the circulatory system. Other disadvantages include the drug itself. It can be irritating to the gastrointestinal tract, it can cause nausea and vomiting, or it can have a bad taste. The most common forms of oral dosages are tablets, capsules, and liquids. See Table 1–5 for dosage forms.

The parenteral routes avoid all the variable conditions that can be present in the gastrointestinal tract and the numerous membrane barriers. For these reasons, more predictable therapeutic blood levels can be achieved quickly. The disadvantage of this mode of administration is once the drug is administered it is virtually irretrievable. Giving a drug by injection usually requires skilled personnel who must be familiar with aseptic technique to avoid introducing bacteria into the patient's system. It is also an expensive means of giving medication. Some of the drugs that are given intravenously can be highly irritating to veins and can cause phlebitis. Other drugs are extravasational and can cause tissue necrosis if they infiltrate. Drugs administered intramuscularly are often painful and irritating to the surrounding tissue and can cause sterile abscesses. Nevertheless, when rapid therapeutic blood levels are required quickly the parenteral route, and in particular the IV route, is the route of choice.

OTHER RESPONSIBILITIES

Nurses are involved in taking a drug history from the patient. Information obtained during the interview includes drug and food allergies, present prescription drugs, medications taken in the past 6 months, self-medication with OTC drugs, vitamins, and recreational drugs. If any allergies are reported, the type of reaction should be ascertained. Taking a drug history affords the nurse the opportunity to determine the level of the patient's understanding of his or her existing condition and the importance of current medications. This information should be used to set the tone and level for further interaction with the individual.

Patient education is a responsibility shared by both nurses and pharmacists. For the patient in the hospital setting, this function is more appropriately handled by the nurse. The nurse should formulate a teaching plan that will be implemented at the time of the patient's discharge. The patient should be thoroughly oriented and informed about the medications that will be prescribed. Points of emphasis include name of medication (both generic and trade name), purpose of medication and how it relates to the patient's condition, side and adverse effects that should be reported to a health professional, how often the medication is taken per day, foods and drinks that should be avoided, and length of time of therapy. In those cases in which drug treatment is a lifelong means of management such as in hypertension, congestive heart failure, diabetes, or epilepsy, additional information such as dietary changes, lifestyle changes, aseptic technique for injections, and the importance of follow-up appointments with a health professional should be included. Some of these lifelong conditions may require more extensive education and awareness; in this case names of local organizations and support groups are invaluable. The clearness with which this information is delivered may very well determine the success or failure of the prescribed drug therapy.

As was mentioned previously, there are specific facts the nurse should be familiar with concerning a drug he or she is about to administer. Given the fact that the pharmaceutical field is so rapidly changing and numerous new drugs are becoming available, it is difficult to keep up. For any unfamiliar drug, the nurse should feel comfortable using the reference books available on the unit. The two most commonly encountered references are the Physician's Desk Reference (PDR), and the American Hospital Formulary Service (AHFS). Each reference serves a specific purpose. The information found in the PDR is the same information the drug manufacturer prints in the package insert; on the other hand, the AHFS presents an independent evaluation of a drug. Even though a new edition of each reference is published on a yearly basis, there are numerous new drugs that become available in between times. These drugs probably will not be found in either reference. In this case a call to the Drug Information Office or to the pharmacy is necessary in order to obtain pertinent information.

SUMMARY

It is obvious that the roles and responsibilities nurses have in drug therapy are multifaceted. The nurse must possess knowledge about drugs, skills, and techniques that pertain to their administration, and verbal skills in order to communicate with other health professionals and the patient. The nurse is the last check point before the medication enters the patient's body. The nurse must possess skills of observation in order to be alert to the patient's response, both beneficial and adverse, to the drugs. It is obvious that in no way can the nurse's importance in successful drug therapy be minimized.

=2= Antipsychotic Agents

Antipsychotic agents are used for the management of psychosis, especially schizophrenia. Before the 1950s, there was no drug therapy available for mental disorders. It was accidental that chlorpromazine, which was developed as an antihistamine, was observed to have a calming effect in psychiatric patients during initial clinical trials. Since that time, many drugs that are structurally similar have been synthesized. The chemical groups that these agents belong to are the phenothiazines, the thioxanthenes, the butyrophenones, and a miscellaneous group of agents (Tables 2–1 and 2–2).

Action and Fate. The actions of the antipsychotic agents are quite similar and will be discussed as a group.

There is evidence to suggest that schizophrenia is based on an imbalance of neurotransmitters with an excessive activity of dopaminergic pathways, specifically in the mesolimbic area of the brain. The exact cause of this overactivity is not known; all of these agents block dopamine receptors in the brain. The main difference among the antipsychotic agents is the type and severity of adverse effects.

All of the antipsychotic agents undergo liver metabolism before they are excreted.

Uses. Schizophrenia is the primary indication for these drugs. Other psychiatric conditions that may respond are manic episodes in manic/depressive individuals and Alzheimer's disease. Gilles de la Tourette syndrome is most responsive to treatment with haloperidol.

Many of the antipsychotic agents also have nonpsychiatric indications. Chlorpromazine has strong antiemetic actions and is also indicated in the treatment of intractable hiccups. Some derivatives are used solely for their antiemetic, antihistaminic, and sedative effects. These agents are prochlorpromazine, promethazine, and benzquinamide. Promethazine is often used in conjunction with other central nervous system (CNS) depressant agents for preoperative sedation.

Side and Adverse Effects. The adverse effects of these agents are numerous and varied (Table 2–3). These agents not only block the dopamine receptors in the mesolimbic area of the brain but they also block the dopamine receptors in the nigrostriatal area, cholinergic receptors, alpha adrenergic receptors, and histamine receptors.

Blockade of the dopamine receptors in the nigrostriatal area causes a predominate cholinergic activity initially that is responsible for acute extrapyramidal symptoms. These include a Parkinson's-like syndrome, akathesias (motor restlessness), and acute dystonias (intermittent or sustained spasms). Later, as the dopamine receptors become hypersensitive, a syndrome called tardive dyskinesis (a syndrome consisting of involuntary, hyperkinetic movements) develops. This adverse effect is not reversible even with dosage reduction or discontinuation of

15

TABLE 2–1. ANTIPSYCHOTIC AGENTS

Generic Name	Trade Name(s)	Relative Incidence of Side Effects		
		Extrapyramidal Symptoms	*Sedation*	*Hypotension*
Phenothiazines				
Aliphatic type				
chlorpromazine	Thorazine	+ +	+ + +	+ +
triflupromazine	Vesprin	+ +	+ + +	+ +
Piperazine type				
acetophenazine	Tindal	+ + +	+ +	+
carphenazine	Proketazine	+ + +	+ +	+
fluphenazine	Prolixin, Permitil	+ + +	+	+
perphenazine	Trilafon	+ + +	+	+
prochlorperazine	Compazine	+ + +	+ +	+
trifluoperazine	Stelazine	+ + +	+	+
Piperidine type				
mesoridazine	Serentil	+	+ + +	+ +
piperacetazine	Quide	+	+ +	+
thioridazine	Mellaril	+	+ + +	+ +
Thioxanthenes				
chlorprothixene	Taractan	+ +	+ + +	+ + +
thiothixene	Navane	+ + +	+	+
Butyrophenone				
haloperidol	Haldol	+ + +	+	+
Dibenzoxazepine				
loxapine	Loxitane	+ + +	+ +	+
Dihydroindolone				
molindone	Moban	+ +	+ +	+ +

+ = Minimum effect; + + = intermediate effect; + + + = maximum effect.

the drug, and there is no effective drug treatment for this effect. Dopamine receptor blockade in other parts of the brain causes release of prolactin which causes galactorrhea, gynecomastia, weight gain, and hypothermia. Blockade of the dopamine receptors in the chemoreceptor trigger zone (CTZ) in the medulla exerts an antiemetic effect.

Other side effects include sedation, anticholinergic effects, orthostatic hypotension, allergic reactions, photosensitivity, lower seizure threshold, hypo- or hyperglycemia, retinopathy, blood dyscrasias, and inhibition of ejaculation and impotence in males.

Contraindications and Cautions. Antipsychotic agents should not be used in comatose states. They should not be used in individuals prone to seizures, and they should be used with caution in individuals with hepatic or renal impairment, hypo- or hypertension, or diabetes.

NURSING IMPLICATIONS

- Before initiating treatment with any of the antipsychotic agents, baseline CBCs, blood pressure, and cardiac function should be established.
- Advise patients, especially the elderly, to avoid an abrupt change from lying to standing position.
- Ensure that the patient is swallowing and not hoarding the medication.

TABLE 2–2. LONG-ACTING INTRAMUSCULAR PREPARATIONS

Generic Name	Trade Name
fluphenazine decanoate	Prolixin Decanoate
fluphenazine enanthate	Prolixin Enanthate

TABLE 2–3. SUMMARY OF ADVERSE EFFECTS BY SYSTEMS ASSOCIATED WITH THE USE OF PHENOTHIAZINES

System	Adverse Effects
Immune	Eczema, erythema, itching, photosensitivity, urticaria
Central nervous system	Sedation, drowsiness, dizziness, syncope, insomnia, reduced REM sleep, bizarre dreams, cerebral edema, convulsive seizures, hyperpyrexia, inability to sweat, depressed cough reflex, catatonic-like states, psychotic symptoms, extrapyramidal symptoms (EPS)[a], EEG changes
Cardiovascular	Orthostatic hypotension, hypertension, palpitations, tachycardia, bradycardia, ECG changes (prolonged QT and PR intervals, blunting of T waves, and ST depression)
Dermatologic	Urticaria, contact dermatitis, exfoliate dermatitis, photosensitivity with cutaneous blue-gray pigmentation, hirsutism (long-term use)
Gastrointestinal	Oral syndrome (xerostomia, vesicular lesions on tongue and mucous membranes, cheilitis, white or black furry tongue, glossitis), constipation, adynamic ileus, cholestatic jaundice, aggravation of peptic ulcers, dyspepsia, increased appetite
Hematologic	Agranulocytosis, thrombocytopenia, purpura, pancytopenia (rare), anemia
Ophthalmic	Blurred vision, increased intraocular pressure, opacity of the lens, mydriasis, miosis, photophobia
Reproductive and genitourinary	Anovulation, infertility, pseudopregnancy, menstrual irregularities, gynecomastia (both sexes), galactorrhea, inhibition of ejaculation, reduced libido, urinary retention or frequency
Respiratory	Nasal congestion, laryngospasm, bronchospasm, respiratory depression
Other	Hypoglycemia, hyperglycemia, enlarged parotid glands, peripheral edema, anaphalactoid reactions, SLE-like syndrome, sudden unexplained death

[a] Pseudoparkinsonism, dystonias, akathisia, tardive dyskinesia.

- Monitor bowel elimination and urinary output.
- Patient may complain of being cold and may need additional cover. Monitor temperature of shower or bath; patient may scald self due to hypothermia.
- Patients should avoid direct exposure to sunlight.
- Diabetics should closely monitor blood and urine glucose levels.
- Antipsychotic agents cause marked CNS depression.
- Abrupt discontinuation of drug is associated with severe gastrointestinal upset and onset of acute extrapyramidal systems.
- Patients may be noncompliant due to extrapyramidal or anticholinergic side effects. Males may avoid medication because of impotence or inhibition of ejaculation.
- Be familiar with the extrapyramidal side effects associated with antipsychotic medications:

    Pseudoparkinsonism: Slowing of voluntary movements, mask facies, rigidity, tremor, and pill-rolling motion.
    Acute dystonia: Abnormal posturing, grimacing, spastic torticollis, and oculogyric crisis.
    Akathisia: Inability to sit still.
    Tardive dyskinesia: Involuntary rhythmic, bizarre movements of face, jaw, mouth, and tongue. Usually irreversible; early detection and discontinuation of drug may reverse symptoms.

Review Questions

1. It is thought that schizophrenia is based on an imbalance of neurotransmitters with an excessive activity of:
   a. acetylcholine
   b. gamma-aminobutyric acid (GABA)
   c. norepinephrine
   d. dopamine

2. Explain why antipsychotic agents induce a Parkinson's-like syndrome.

3. Define:
   a. Akathisia
   b. Acute dystonia
   c. Tardive dyskinesia

4–10. Matching: Choose the statement in column B that best describes each drug in column A.

Column A	Column B
4. ＿＿＿＿ Thorazine	a. High incidence of extrapyramidal symptoms
5. ＿＿＿＿ Stelazine	b. High incidence of sedation
6. ＿＿＿＿ Mellaril	
7. ＿＿＿＿ Navane	
8. ＿＿＿＿ Haldol	
9. ＿＿＿＿ Compazine	
10. ＿＿＿＿ Prolixin	

11. Gilles de la Tourette syndrome is usually treated with:
    a. Mellaril
    b. Haldol
    c. Stelazine
    d. Loxitane

12. Individuals experiencing intractable hiccoughs may be treated with:
    a. chlorpromazine
    b. trifluperazine
    c. molindone
    d. thioridazine

13. Phenothiazines are more likely to cause:
    a. hypertension
    b. hypotension

14. Phenothiazines are more likely to:
    a. raise seizure threshold
    b. lower seizure threshold

15. It is not unusual for patients taking antipsychotic agents to experience:
    a. hypothermia
    b. hyperthermia

16. Tardive dyskinesia:
    a. has an early onset
    b. is usually irreversible
    c. may be treated with anticholinergic agents
    d. disappears when drug is discontinued

17. Phenothiazines may cause:
    a. hypoglycemia
    b. hyperglycemia

c. either

d. neither

18. Patients taking antipsychotic agents frequently experience:

a. sedation

b. constipation

c. syncope

d. all of the above

19–30. Matching:

Generic Name	**Trade Name**
19. _____ thioridazine	a. Navane
20. _____ thiothixene	b. Stelazine
21. _____ haloperidol	c. Compazine
22. _____ chlorpromazine	d. Prolixin
23. _____ trifluperazine	e. Loxitane
24. _____ triflupromazine	f. Thorazine
25. _____ prochlorperazine	g. Trilafon
26. _____ fluphenazine	h. Mobane
27. _____ perphenazine	i. Mellaril
28. _____ molindone	j. Vesprin
29. _____ loxapine	k. Taractan
30. _____ chlorprothixene	l. Haldol

=3=
Antidepressants and Lithium

Depression is a heterogeneous disorder characterized by fatigue, musculoskeletal complaints, sleep disorders, a loss of joy of living, and guilt. Based on origin, depression may be classified as (1) "reactive" or "secondary" depression (60 percent of cases) which occurs in response to some exogenous situation (grief, illness, loss of job); (2) "endogenous" depression (25 percent of cases), which is thought to be genetic in nature; and (3) depression associated with bipolar (manic/depressive) affective disorder (10 to 15 percent of cases). The drugs discussed in this section are used to treat the second and third types of depression.

Depression, like schizophrenia, is thought to have a biochemical basis. In this case, however, there is a deficiency or a decreased functioning most probably of the neurotransmitters norepinephrine and serotonin. The physiological basis for the bipolar affective disorder is less clear.

The drugs discussed in this section are used primarily to treat endogeneous depression and the bipolar affective disorders (Table 3–1). The management of endogeneous depression is with the tricyclic antidepressant agents (TCAs) and related compounds and the monoamine oxidase inhibitors (MAOIs). For the bipolar affective disorder, the drug used to stabilize mood alterations is lithium carbonate.

Tricyclic Antidepressant Agents (TCAs)

Action and Fate. TCAs block the re-uptake pump for serotonin and norepinephrine. This action increases the concentration of these two transmitters in the synaptic cleft and allows them to remain there for a longer period of time.

Most of the tricyclics are metabolized in the liver to active metabolites which must undergo further biotransformation in order to be excreted via the urine.

Uses. The major indication for these agents is to treat endogenous depression. An additional use for imipramine is for the control of enuresis.

Side and Adverse Effects. The more common side effects of TCAs are due to their anticholinergic and alpha receptor blocking effects. These blocking effects cause dry mouth, blurred vision, urinary retention, constipation, tachycardia, sedation, and hypotension. Central nervous system (CNS) side effects include tremor, speech blockage, and a paradoxical anxiety and insomnia. These agents also lower seizure threshold.

Contraindications and Cautions. The use of TCAs is contraindicated during the acute recovery phase following a myocardial infarction: these agents may precipitate arrhythmias. Use with caution in patients with a history of seizure disorder, urinary retention, glaucoma, or cardiovascular disorder.

TABLE 3–1. ANTIDEPRESSANTS AND LITHIUM

Generic Name	Trade Name(s)	Sedative Activity	Anticholinergic Activity	Adult Daily Dose Range (mg)
Antidepressants				
Tricyclic compounds				
desipramine	Norpramin Pertofrane	+	+	75–150
imipramine	Tofranil	+ +	+ +	75–150
trimipramine	Surmontil	+ + +	+ +	75–150
amitriptyline	Elavil Endep	+ + +	+ + +	75–150
protriptyline	Vivactil	+	+ +	15–40
nortriptyline	Aventyl Pamelor	+ +	+	20–100
doxepin	Adapin Sinequan	+ + +	+ + +	75–150
amoxapine	Asendin	+	+	75–400
Tetracyclic compounds				
maprotiline	Ludiomil	+ +	+ +	75–150
triazolopyridine	—	—	—	—
trazodone	Desyrel	+ +	+	75–300
Monoamine oxidase inhibitors				
isocarboxazid	Marplan	—	—	20–40
phenelzine	Nardil	—	—	45–120
tranylcypromine	Parnate	—	—	10–20
Antimanic agent				
lithium	Eskalith Lithane Lithobane Lithotabs	—	—	600–2100 (initially) 900–1200 (maintenance)

+ = minimum effect; + + = intermediate effect; + + + = maximum effect.

NURSING IMPLICATIONS

- TCAs have a slow onset of action (3 to 4 weeks).
- Monitor blood pressure and pulse for irregularities in patient's heart rate. Twice yearly ECG is advised for patients with cardiovascular disease.
- Suicide is a risk with depressed patients. Ensure patient is not hoarding medication.
- Warn patient about sedative effects of medication. Once a day, dose may be administered at bedtime.
- Dry mouth may be relieved by sucking on hard candy.
- Patient may require stool softener to relieve constipation.
- Alcohol will potentiate CNS depression.
- Caution patient regarding orthostatic hypotension.

Monoamine Oxidase Inhibitors (MAOIs)

Action and Fate. These agents block the action of the enzyme monoamine oxidase, an intraneuronal enzyme (see Fig. 1–4). This action increases the concentration of norepinephrine and serotonin at the synaptic cleft.

All MAOIs are metabolized in the liver and excreted in the urine.

TABLE 3–2. SYMPTOMS ASSOCIATED WITH HYPERTENSIVE CRISIS

Prodromal symptoms:	Headache and palpitations
Other symptoms include:	Nausea and vomiting
	Dilated pupils
	Sweating
	Bradycardia and tachycardia
	Stiff or sore neck

TABLE 3–3. TYRAMINE-CONTAINING FOODS AND BEVERAGES

Aged meats	Licorice
Avocados	Liver
Bananas	Meat tenderizers
Beer	Pickled or kippered herring
Broad bean pods	Raisins
Canned figs	Sour cream
Cheese	Soy sauce
Chianti and other red wines	Yeast and meat extracts
Chocolate	Yogurt
Cream	

Uses. These agents are used to treat depression in patients not responding or intolerant to TCAs.

Side and Adverse Effects. The most frequent side effects associated with MAOIs are drowsiness, dry mouth, orthostatic hypotension, blurred vision, dysuria, and constipation.

An important disadvantage of these agents is the dietary restrictions that must be closely followed in order to prevent a hypertensive crisis from occurring. Individuals should avoid tyramine-containing foods such as cheese, avocados, red wine, and beer. In addition, sympathomimetic drugs should also be avoided. The following symptoms could indicate that the patient was having a hypertensive crisis: headache, tachycardia, palpitations, nausea, vomiting, and hypertension.

Contraindications and Cautions. The use of these agents is contraindicated in patients with pheochromocytoma, congestive heart failure, severely impaired renal or liver function, and in patients over 60.

NURSING IMPLICATIONS

• Patient's blood pressure should be monitored frequently to detect any early increase.
• Patient should notify physician if headache or palpitations are experienced, may indicate impending hypertensive crisis (Table 3–2).
• Patient should understand the hazard of ingesting food and beverages containing tyramine (Table 3–3).

Lithium

Action and Fate. The antimanic agent lithium prevents mood swing in those individuals with bipolar affective disorder. The mechanism by which lithium accomplishes this is unknown. Lithium is excreted unchanged in the urine.

Uses. Lithium is used for bipolar affective disorder management.

Side and Adverse Effects. There are many side effects associated with the use of lithium. These include nausea, diarrhea, malaise, and fine hand tremor. See Table 3–4 for symptoms associated with toxic levels of lithium.

Contraindications and Cautions. Lithium is contraindicated in individuals with significant cardiovascular or renal disease, dehydration or sodium depletion, or who are on a low salt diet or sodium-depleting diuretics. Pregnant women should also avoid lithium.

TABLE 3–4. ADVERSE REACTIONS ASSOCIATED WITH TOXIC LEVELS OF LITHIUM

Lithium Level (mEq/L)	Adverse Reactions
1.5–2	Nausea, diarrhea, malaise, fine hand tremor, polyuria, polydipsia, fatigue
2–2.5	Anorexia, nausea, vomiting, blurred vision, motor abnormalities, circulatory collapse, coma
Above 2.5	Generalized convulsions, oliguria, death

NURSING IMPLICATIONS

• Watch for early symptoms of toxicity.
• Emphasize importance of quarterly blood level determinations of lithium. (Therapeutic range is 1.0 to 1.5 mEq/L in acute mania and 0.6 to 1.6 mEq/L for maintenance.)
• Teach the patient to avoid use of diuretics that cause increased sodium excretion such as the thiazide and loop diuretics. Excessive sodium excretion causes lithium retention, which may lead to toxic levels.

Review Questions

List the three types of depression.

1. _____
2. _____
3. _____

The proposed biochemical basis of endogenous depression is caused by deficiencies of which two neurotransmitters?

4. _____
5. _____

6. Which one of the following antidepressants may also be used to control enuresis?
   a. imipramine
   b. desipramine
   c. amitriptyline
   d. nortriptyline

7. Tricyclic antidepressants often are administered at bedtime due to their _____ effect.
   a. sympathomimetic
   b. hypotensive
   c. sedative
   d. anticholinergic

8. Tricyclic antidepressants should be used with caution in patients with:
   a. seizure disorders
   b. glaucoma
   c. cardiovascular disorders
   d. all of the above

List six foods that contain tyramine.

9. _____

10. _____

11. _____

12. _____

13. _____

14. _____

15. Patients who ingest tyramine-containing foods while taking monoamine oxidase inhibitors will experience:
    a. severe drop in blood pressure
    b. severe rise in blood pressure
    c. a pronounced cholinergic reaction
    d. a pronounced anticholinergic reaction

16. Give the primary indication for the use of lithium carbonate.

17. Drugs such as the thiazide and loop diuretics should be avoided in individuals taking lithium because they cause an:
    a. abnormal retention of lithium
    b. excessive loss of lithium

Give four adverse reactions associated with toxic levels of lithium.

18. _____

19. _____

20. _____

21. _____

22–30. Matching:

Generic Name	**Trade Name**
22. _____ desipramine	a. Parnate
23. _____ trazodone	b. Marplan
24. _____ lithium	c. Adapin
25. _____ isocarboxazide	d. Vivactil
26. _____ doxepin	e. Elavil
27. _____ imipramine	f. Tofranil
28. _____ protriptyline	g. Norpramine
29. _____ amitriptyline	h. Eskalith
30. _____ tranylcypromine	i. Desyrel

=4=

Antianxiety and Hypnotic Agents

Agents classified as antianxiety or hypnotic agents are all classed as central nervous system (CNS) depressants. Antianxiety medications (formerly called sedatives) are used to calm an individual or decrease his or her anxiety level. A hypnotic, on the other hand, is used to induce sleep by causing a greater degree of CNS depression. Some of the agents are classed solely as hypnotic agents (e.g., flurazepam), others can be classed as either an antianxiety agent or hypnotic (e.g., diazepam). The desired effect of these latter agents can be produced by simply using a lower or higher dose.

The agents discussed in this unit fall in one of three classes: the benzodiazepines, the barbiturates, and a miscellaneous group.

BENZODIAZEPINES

The first benzodiazepine, chlordiazepoxide, was introduced in 1960. Since then numerous other benzodiazepines have been developed (Table 4–1). For the most part they have replaced the barbiturates as antianxiety agents and hypnotics because of their greater margin of safety, less addicting potential, and lack of effect on the microsomal enzymes. In addition, used as hypnotics the benzodiazepines induce a more natural sleep with more time spent in REM.

Action and Fate. The benzodiazepines act on the limbic system in the brain to reduce anxiety. The exact mechanism by which they do this is unclear but there is some evidence that they potentiate the actions of the inhibitory neurotransmitter gamma-aminobutyric acid (GABA).

Once absorbed systemically, the fate is agent dependent. Table 4–1 summarizes the metabolic fate and half-lives of the various benzodiazepines and Figure 4–1 gives the interrelationship of several of the benzodiazepines.

Uses. The benzodiazepines are used to treat anxiety disorders. They are recommended for severe, immobilizing anxiety, and panic disorders. These agents are also used as hypnotics to treat insomnia.

In addition, chlordiazepoxide oxazepam, and diazepam are used to treat symptoms associated with alcohol withdrawal and diazepam is considered one of the drugs of choice for status epilepticus.

Side and Adverse Effects. The major adverse effect of the benzodiazepines is CNS depression characterized by drowsiness, sluggishness, and impaired motor coordination. The elderly are especially prone to paradoxical excitation, confusion, disorientation, and ataxia. Psychological dependence and physiological dependence can both occur with the benzodiazepines.

TABLE 4–1. VARIOUS BENZODIAZEPINE PREPARATIONS

Generic Name	Trade Names (Control Substance Schedule)	Major Therapeutic Indications	Major Active Metabolite(s)	Half-life ($t_{1/2}$) (hr)
alprazolam	Xanax (CIV)	Anxiety, anxiety with depression	desmethyldiazepam	50–100
chlorazepate	Tranxene (CIV)	Anxiety	desmethyldiazepam	50–100
chlordiazepoxide	Librium (CIV)	Anxiety, preoperative sedation, symptoms associated with alcohol withdrawal	desmethylchlordiazepoxide	24–96 8–24[a]
diazepam	Valium (CIV)	Anxiety, preoperative sedation, muscle spasm, symptoms associated with alcohol withdrawal, status epilepticus	desmethyldiazepam	50–100 27–37[a]
flurazepam	Dalmane (CIV)	Insomnia	desalkylflurazepam	74–160
lorazepam	Ativan (CIV)	Anxiety, preoperative sedation	None	8–25
oxazepam	Serax (CIV)	Anxiety, symptoms associated with alcohol withdrawal	None	5–15
prazepam	Centrax (CIV) Verstran (CIV)	Anxiety	desmethyldiazepam	50–100
temazepam	Restoril (CIV)	Insomnia	None	8–38
triazolam	Halcion (CIV)	Insomnia	None	2–5

[a] Indicates half-life of therapeutically active parent compound.

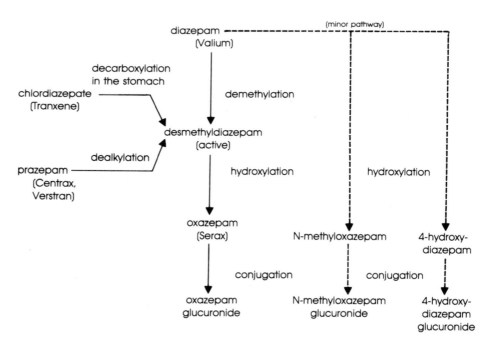

Figure 4–1. Diagrammatic scheme of the metabolic inter-relationship of several benzodiazepines.

Contraindications and Cautions. The use of these agents is contraindicated in individuals with glaucoma or myasthenia gravis. Selection of the appropriate agent is based on the age and pathological status of the patient. Benzodiazepines with long half-lives and many active metabolites should be given in lower doses or completely avoided in the elderly and those individuals with impaired liver or renal function. Benzodiazepines should be used cautiously with other CNS depressants such as alcohol, opioids, tricyclic antidepressants, and other antianxiety or hypnotic agents.

NURSING IMPLICATIONS

In most instances, the patient will be self-medicating with these agents. However, there are certain areas that the nurse can be helpful in instructing the patient in the proper use of these medications.

- Warn the individual not to consume alcohol and other CNS depressants.
- Instruct the individual to take the drug as prescribed and not to modify the dose or dosing interval.
- Caution individuals against activities that require motor coordination such as driving or operating machinery.
- It is especially important to take precautions with the elderly after administering a dose. They should be located where they are not prone to fall and they should be assisted if ambulating.
- Evaluate the patient for reduced anxiety. Parameters such as blood pressure, pulse rate, and respirations should be compared to baseline values.
- Evaluate quality of sleep for hypnotics. Note complaints of "sleep hangover," a condition that occurs if an individual is not experiencing enough REM sleep.
- All benzodiazepines are controlled substances with abuse and psychological and physiological addicting potential.

BARBITURATES

Before the introduction of the benzodiazepines, the barbiturates (Table 4–2) were the mainstay of drug treatment for anxiety and insomnia. Now, by and large, they have been replaced by the benzodiazepines.

Action and Fate. The barbiturates potentiate the action of the inhibitory neurotransmitter GABA in a way similar to the benzodiazepines.

A portion of two barbiturates, barbital and phenobarbital, is excreted unchanged. The other barbiturates are metabolized in the liver to inactive metabolites that are then excreted via the urine.

TABLE 4–2. BARBITURATES

Generic Name	Trade Name	Duration of Action	Use	Schedule
Ultrashort-acting agents				
thiopental	Pentothal	20–30 min	Anesthetic	CIII
Short- to intermediate-acting agents				
amobarbital	Amytal	6–11 hr	Sedative/hypnotic	CII
butabarbital	Butisol	6–11 hr	Sedative/hypnotic	CIII
pentobarbital	Nembutal	3–6 hr	Sedative/hypnotic	CII
secobarbital	Seconal	3–6 hr	Sedative/hypnotic	CII
Long-acting agents				
mephobarbital	Mebaral	8–16 hr	Anticonvulsive	CIV
methabarbital	Gemonil	8–16 hr	Anticonvulsive	CIII
phenobarbital	Luminal	8–16 hr	Anticonvulsive	CIV

TABLE 4–3. MISCELLANEOUS HYPNOTICS

Generic Name	Trade Name	Schedule
chloral hydrate	Noctec	CIV
paraldehyde	—	CIV
ethchlorvynol	Placidyl	CIV
glutethimide	Doriden	CIII
methylprylon	Noludar	CIII

Uses. The use of short- to intermediate-acting agents is limited to hypnosis. The ultrashort acting thiopental is used as an adjunct to anesthesia. The long-acting barbiturates are used as anticonvulsants (see Chapter 7).

Side and Adverse Effects. CNS depression is a major problem of the barbiturates, which cause drowsiness, confusion, and lack of motor coordination. The elderly are especially susceptible to this effect.

The barbiturates and, in particular, phenobarbital, cause an induction of the microsomal enzymes. These are the enzymes located in the liver that are involved in the metabolism of drugs. Stimulation of these enzymes can decrease the duration of action and therapeutic effects of many other drugs.

Certain patients will experience a paradoxical excitation with barbiturates. This seems to happen more often in children and elderly.

The margin of safety of the barbiturates is very narrow, therefore, an overdose can cause fatal respiratory depression. Physiological addiction to barbiturates is a very serious consequence. Individuals who are addicted must be tapered off slowly. Abrupt discontinuation of barbiturates causes delirium, convulsions, or death.

Contraindications and Cautions. Barbiturates should not be used in individuals who are mentally depressed or have respiratory depression. They should be used cautiously in patients with impaired liver failure.

NURSING IMPLICATIONS

The same guidelines for the benzodiazepines apply to the barbiturates. In addition, it is important for the nurse to emphasize that barbiturates should not be abruptly discontinued. All barbiturates are controlled substances with abuse and psychological and physiological addicting potential.

MISCELLANEOUS HYPNOTIC AGENTS

This third class of agents (Table 4–3) shares many common characteristics with the benzodiazepines and barbiturates. All of these agents can cause both psychological and physiological dependence. Of all the agents listed in this class, chloral hydrate is probably the most frequently used. It is used as a hypnotic in the elderly and in children especially and as a sedative in children prior to certain procedures. Because the use of these agents has declined, no further discussion will be given and the reader is referred to a pharmacology textbook for more information.

Review Questions

Give four reasons why the benzodiazepines have replaced the barbiturates as antianxiety and hypnotic agents.

1. _____

2. _____

3. _____

4. _____

5–11. Matching: (Answers may be used more than once.)

Drug	**Use**
5. ____ chlordiazepoxide	a. used in alcohol withdrawal
6. ____ triazolam	b. used in anxious individuals with
7. ____ oxazepam	depression
8. ____ lorazepam	c. used for muscle spasm
9. ____ diazepam	d. used only for insomnia
10. ____ flurazepam	e. may be used for preoperative seda-
11. ____ temazepam	tion

12. A rational choice for anxiety in an elderly individual would be:
    a. diazepam
    b. chlordiazepoxide
    c. chlorazepate
    d. oxazepam

13. All benzodiazepines are classed as _____ controlled substances.
    a. CII
    b. CIII
    c. CIV
    d. CV

14–18. Matching:

Drug	**Duration of Action**
14. ____ phenobarbital	a. ultra-short-acting barbiturates
15. ____ secobarbital	b. short- to intermediate-acting barbitu-
16. ____ thiopental	rates
17. ____ pentobarbital	c. long-acting barbiturates
18. ____ methabarbital	

19. Both the benzodiazepines and the barbiturates act by potentiating which neurotransmitter?
    a. Gamma-aminobutyric acid (GABA)
    b. Acetylcholine
    c. Serotonin
    d. Dopamine

20. The barbiturates can alter the duration of action of certain drugs by:
    a. stimulating the microsomal enzyme activity
    b. inhibiting the microsomal enzyme activity

21. Among the signs and symptoms of barbiturate poisoning is:
    a. hypertension
    b. arrhythmias
    c. respiratory alkalosis
    d. respiratory depression

22. Which one of the following sedatives or hypnotics is frequently used in pediatrics?
    a. glutethimide
    b. ethchlorvynol
    c. methylprylon
    d. chloral hydrate

=5=

Central Nervous System Stimulants and Anorectics

In recent years, the use of central nervous system (CNS) agents has been limited because of their abuse potential and serious adverse effects. The agents discussed in this section are the amphetamines, methylphenidate, cocaine, and the anorectic agents (Table 5–1).

Action and Fate. The amphetamines are a group of agents that share a common basic structure and pharmacological properties. They are synthetic sympathomimetics with both alpha and beta adrenergic receptor activity. These agents act directly on adrenergic receptors by (1) increasing the release of norepinephrine and dopamine from CNS neurons and (2) blocking the re-uptake of these neurotransmitters. The amphetamines are primarily excreted unchanged via the urine. They will cross the placenta and are found in breast milk.

Methylphenidate is pharmacologically related to the amphetamines but it is a less potent CNS stimulant. Its exact mechanism of action, however, has not been determined. The drug is metabolized in the body and the metabolites excreted in the urine. Safe use during pregnancy has not been established.

Cocaine is an alkaloid obtained from the leaves of the *Erythroxylon coca* plant. If applied topically, it blocks nerve conduction producing local anesthesia and vasoconstriction. Systemically, cocaine produces an adrenergic effect by acting as an indirect sympathomimetic agent. It exerts its adrenergic action by blocking the neuronal re-uptake of epinephrine and norepinephrine. Cocaine is readily absorbed through mucous membranes. It is metabolized in the liver and excreted primarily as metabolites in the urine.

The anorectics are structurally and pharmacologically related to the amphetamines, with a similar mechanism of action. Their safe use during pregnancy has not been established.

Uses. The amphetamines are used to treat narcolepsy, hyperactivity in children with minimal brain damage, and as short-term aids in weight reduction. Amphetamines can also produce behavioral changes such as increased alertness and euphoria.

Methylphenidate is indicated for narcolepsy and hyperactivity in children but not as an appetite suppressant. It apparently improves motor ability, mood, and mental function without the effects on the peripheral circulatory system seen with the amphetamines.

The use of cocaine is limited to topical anesthesia of the eye and nasal sinuses. It may be included in some formulations of Brompton's cocktail.

TABLE 5–1. CENTRAL NERVOUS SYSTEM STIMULANTS AND ANORECTIC AGENTS

Generic Name	Trade Name	Controlled Substance Class
Amphetamines		
amphetamine complex	Biphetamine	CII
amphetamine	Benzedrine	CII
dextroamphetamine	Dexedrine	CII
methamphetamine	Desoxyn	CII
Nonamphetamines		
cocaine	—	CII
methylphenidate	Ritalin	CII
Anorectic agents		
benzphetamine	Didrex	CIII
chlorphentermine	Pre-Sate	CIII
diethylpropion	Tenuate, Tepanil	CIV
fenfluramine	Pondimin	CIV
mazindol	Sanorex	CIV
phendimetrazine	Bontril, Plegine	CIII
phenmetrazine	Preludin	CII
phentermine	Adipex-P, Fastin, Ionamin	CIV

The use of anorectics is indicated in the short-term management of obesity in conjunction with proper diet modifications.

Side and Adverse Effects. All of these agents will produce in varying degrees anorexia, insomnia, headache, nervousness, increased blood pressure, and pulse changes. They can worsen or precipitate angina, cardiac arrhythmias, and congestive heart failure. In addition, prolonged topical application of cocaine to the nasal mucosa will cause perforation of the nasal system. Systemic absorption of cocaine causes CNS stimulation: insomnia, anorexia, euphoria, excitation, nervousness, and heart arrhythmias that can cause sudden death. Tolerance and physiological and psychological addiction can occur to all these agents.

Contraindications and Cautions. Any hypersensitivity reaction to the agent is a contraindication for its use. These agents should not be used for normal fatigue states, or in individuals with seizure disorders, cardiovascular disorders, glaucoma, anxiety, tension, agitation, or severe depression. Close monitoring of individuals who are prescribed these agents is required. Their use should be limited in those individuals with a history of drug abuse.

NURSING IMPLICATIONS

- Closely monitor blood pressure, pulse, and cardiac status in patient taking these drugs and compare to baseline values.
- These agents should be administered before 6 PM to avoid insomnia.
- It is important to monitor the weight in children taking amphetamines or methylphenidate for hyperactivity, in order to ascertain weight reduction.
- Discontinuation of these agents leads to a period of severe mental depression. The patient should be closely observed for indications of potential suicide attempts during this time period.
- Cocaine used as a throat anesthetic can cause temporary paralysis of the respiratory cilia. Patients should be advised not to take anything by mouth until sensation returns in order to avoid aspiration.
- All these drugs are controlled substances with abuse, physiological, and psychological addicting potential. Refer to Table 5–1 for control schedule for individual agents.

Review Questions

1. The anorectics are related to:
   a. amphetamines
   b. cocaine
   c. methylphenidate
   d. none of the above

2. Which one of the following agents is preferred in treating hyperactive children?
   a. Desoxyn
   b. Dexedrine
   c. Ritalin
   d. Ionamin

3. What is the current accepted medical use of cocaine?
   a. to relieve nasal congestion
   b. as a mood elevator
   c. as a prophylactic agent for excessive bleeding prior to rhinoplasty
   d. as a topical anesthetic

4. The major ingredient in most nonprescription appetite suppressants is:
   a. benzocaine
   b. phenylpropanolamine
   c. methylcellulose
   d. caffeine

5. All of the following may be adverse effects of amphetamine-like anorectic drugs except:
   a. low blood pressure
   b. headache
   c. insomnia
   d. constipation

6. Amphetamine-like anorectic drugs are generally contraindicated in all of the following medical conditions except:
   a. hypertension
   b. asthma
   c. angina pectoris
   d. hyperthyroidism

7. Give the mechanism of action of amphetamine.

8. Give the mechanism of action of cocaine.

9–18. Fill in the missing information:

Generic Name	Trade Name	Controlled Substance Class
9. _____	Biphetamine	_____
10. amphetamine	_____	_____
11. dextroamphetamine	_____	_____
12. cocaine	_____	_____
13. _____	Ritalin	_____
14. _____	Didrex	_____
15. _____	Pre-Sate	_____
16. diethylpropion	_____	_____
17. phenmetrazine	_____	_____
18. _____	Ionamin	_____

=6= Antiparkinsonism Agents

Parkinson's disease results from a deficiency of dopamine within the striatum of the brain. This deficiency causes an imbalance between dopamine, an inhibitory neurotransmitter, and acetylcholine, an excitatory neurotransmitter. The disease is characterized by extrapyramidal movements, tremor, akinesia, and rigidity. In addition to drugs, the treatment regimen includes physiotherapy, exercise, and psychological support. Drug therapy attempts to restore the normal balance by increasing dopamine levels in the brain and inhibiting cholinergic system dominance with anticholinergic drugs.

In advanced stages of the disease, patients literally become frozen and are unable to care for themselves. This loss of motor function accounts for impaired postural reflexes, reduced blinking, mask-like facies, and ocular convergence. Also common are sialorrhea (an excessive secretion of saliva), seborrhea (overactive sebaceous glands), and hyperhidrosis (excessive sweating).

ANTICHOLINERGIC AND ANTICHOLINERGIC-LIKE AGENTS

All the drugs listed in Table 6–1 as anticholinergic and anticholinergic-like agents will be considered as a group in this section. These agents are not as effective as the dopamine-restoring agents but they are useful in those individuals with mild parkinsonism. These agents may also be used in combination with the dopamine-restoring agents.

Action and Fate. The antiparkinsonism effect of these agents appears to be related to their central anticholinergic properties. They reduce the cholinergic dominance, thus diminishing symptoms such as akinesia, rigidity, and tremor. They also improve other symptoms such as depressed mood, and excessive salivation and sweating.

Use. These agents are used in individuals who have mild Parkinson's disease or in conjunction with the other agents that increase dopamine activity in the brain.

Side and Adverse Effects. Most commonly these agents cause dry mouth, mydriasis, cycloplegia, tachycardia, constipation, urinary retention. Paradoxical hyperexcitation may occur in the elderly.

Contraindications and Cautions. These agents should be used cautiously in patients with gastrointestinal disturbance or prostatic hypertrophy. They may also precipitate a glaucoma attack in predisposed patients.

37

TABLE 6–1. DRUGS USED TO TREAT PARKINSON'S DISEASE

Generic Name	Trade Name
Anticholinergic agents	
benztropine	Cogentin
biperiden	Akineton
cycrimine	Pagitane
procyclidine	Kemadrin
trihexyphenidyl	Artane
Anticholinergic-like agents	
diphenhydramine	Benadryl
ethopropazine	Parsidol
Dopamine-releasing agent	
amantadine	Symmetrel
Agents that increase brain levels of dopamine (dopamine replacement agents)	
levodopa	Dopar, Larodopa
levodopa/carbidopa	Sinemet
Dopamine agonist	
bromocriptine	Parlodel

NURSING IMPLICATIONS

- Caution patient about drowsiness and blurred vision. Other central nervous system (CNS) depressants and alcohol will enhance drowsiness.
- Dry mouth may be relieved with hard candy or sugarless gum.
- The diminished sweating is hazardous in summer. Caution patient to avoid strenuous activity in heat.
- Patients may require a stool softener to manage constipation that occurs.
- Monitor input-output ratios to determine if urinary retention is occurring. Especially important in those with prostatic hypertrophy.

DRUGS THAT AFFECT DOPAMINE LEVEL IN THE BRAIN

Amantadine

Action and Fate. Amantadine increases the concentration of dopamine in the brain by either increasing its synthesis, inhibiting its re-uptake, or stimulating its release from storage vesicles. It is excreted unchanged in the urine.

Use. Amantadine was developed originally as an antiviral agent (see Chapter 16 under Antiviral Agents) that was accidentally discovered to improve symptoms associated with Parkinson's disease.

Side and Adverse Effects. Patients taking amantadine may experience hallucinations, confusion, or nightmares. Other adverse effects include lethargy, drowsiness, slurred speech, insomnia, and orthostatic hypotension.

Amantadine has several CNS side effects. These include restlessness, depression, excitation, and confusion. Another side effect that is relatively common is livedo reticularis, a purplish discoloration of the skin. Peripheral edema, orthostatic hypotension, and congestive heart failure also occur.

Contraindications and Cautions. This drug should be used cautiously in individuals who have a history of seizures or congestive heart failure.

NURSING IMPLICATIONS

- Abrupt discontinuation may cause a parkinsonism crisis.
- Advise patient to change positions slowly to avoid falling due to orthostatic hypotension.

Levodopa and Levodopa/Carbidopa

Action and Fate. Dopamine itself does not penetrate the blood–brain barrier; for this reason it would be of no value in the treatment of Parkinson's disease. The precursor of dopamine, levodopa, does however penetrate the blood–brain barrier and is enzymatically converted in the brain to dopamine. The combination of levodopa and carbidopa was formulated to prevent degradation of levodopa by an enzyme found in peripheral tissue, increasing the amount of levodopa available to enter the brain.

Levodopa is converted to dopamine which is rapidly metabolized and excreted in the urine.

Use. Levodopa is used in the management of Parkinson's disease.

Side and Adverse Effects. Nausea, vomiting, and anorexia occur in most individuals initially, especially if the dose of levodopa is large. These gastrointestinal disturbances are lessened if levodopa is combined with carbidopa. A variety of arrhythmias have been reported also. Other cardiovascular effects include orthostatic hypotension. Abnormal involuntary movements may develop in individuals who have taken levodopa for a long time.

Contraindications and Cautions. Use contraindicated in narrow angle glaucoma, acute psychosis, or severe psychoneurosis. Used cautiously in individuals with pre-existing cardiac arrhythmias.

NURSING IMPLICATIONS

- Pyridoxine (vitamin B_6) rapidly reverses therapeutic effect of levodopa because it is a cofactor in its conversion to dopamine.
- Advise patient to take this medication with food to decrease gastrointestinal disturbances.
- Monitor vital signs, especially during initial dosage adjustment period.
- Advise patient that urine and sweat may become darker in color.
- Diabetic patients should be closely monitored for alterations in blood sugar control.
- Levodopa and phenothiazines are mutually antagonistic. Levodopa may enhance hypotensive effects of guanethidine and methyldopa.

Bromocriptine

Action and Fate. Bromocriptine is a semisynthetic ergot derivative that acts as a dopamine receptor agonist. It is extensively metabolized in the liver and the majority of the metabolites are excreted in the bile. A minimal amount of drug is excreted unchanged in the urine.

Uses. The use of bromocriptine is indicated in the management of Parkinson's disease if the patient is unresponsive to levodopa or it may be used in combination with levodopa. In addition, bromocriptine has also been used to treat certain endocrinologic disorders, specifically hyperprolactinemia.

Side and Adverse Effects. Nausea is the most common adverse effect in patients receiving bromocriptine. Adverse CNS effects of the drug include headache, migraine, dizziness, drowsiness, and fatigue. Bromocriptine also produces postural hypotension and syncope.

Contraindications and Cautions. Bromocriptine is contraindicated in patients who are sensitive to ergot alkaloids or who have severe ischemic heart or peripheral vascular disease. It should be used with caution in those with hepatic or renal function impairment.

NURSING IMPLICATIONS

- Administer drug with food or milk to decrease gastrointestinal disturbance.
- Observe patient for psychotic symptoms.
- Blood pressure should be monitored closely for hypotension initially.
- Advise patient to avoid driving and other activities that require motor coordination.
- Concurrent use of diuretics and phenothiazines with bromocriptine is not recommended. Monitor patient for potentiation of hypotensive effect if taking antihypertensive medication.

Review Questions

1. Parkinson's disease develops as a result of a deficiency of which one of the following neurotransmitters?
   a. Norepinephrine
   b. Acetylcholine
   c. Dopamine
   d. GABA

2. Side effects associated with the use of anticholinergic drugs include:
   a. constipation
   b. urinary retention
   c. sedation
   d. all of the above

3. The simultaneous administration of which vitamin with levodopa decreases its effectiveness?
   a. vitamin C
   b. vitamin B_1
   c. vitamin B_6
   d. vitamin E

4. The patient is advised to take levodopa with food in order to:
   a. reduce gastrointestinal side effects
   b. enhance absorption
   c. prevent enzymatic degradation of the drug
   d. mask the unpleasant taste

List three side effects of amantadine.

5. _____

6. _____

7. _____

Give four physical manifestations of Parkinson's disease.

8. _____

9. _____

10. _____

11. _____

12–17. Matching:

Generic Name	Trade Name
12. ____ benztropine	a. Benadryl
13. ____ levodopa/carbidopa	b. Symmetrel

14. _____ trihexylphenidyl   c. Parlodel
15. _____ amantadine   d. Sinemet
16. _____ diphenhydramine   e. Cogentin
17. _____ bromocriptine   f. Artane

18–25. Matching:

Agent   **Agent Class**

18. _____ Parlodel   a. anticholinergic agent
19. _____ Dopar   b. anticholinergic-like agent
20. _____ Benadryl   c. dopamine-releasing agent
21. _____ Cogentin   d. dopamine replacement agent
22. _____ Kemadrin   e. dopamine agonist
23. _____ Symmetrel
24. _____ Sinemet
25. _____ Artane

26. The anticholinergic and anticholinergic-like drugs are useful in the management of:
   a. urinary retention
   b. decreased visual acuity
   c. confusion
   d. excessive salivation

=7= Anticonvulsant Agents

Anticonvulsant agents (Table 7–1) are used to reduce the number and severity of seizures in individuals with epilepsy. It is estimated that about 1 percent of the population in the United States has epilepsy. Seizures are not a disease but a symptom of some underlying disorder that results from an abnormal transmission in cerebral neurons. In most cases the underlying cause is unknown, i.e., idiopathic. In other cases, seizures may also be due to high fever, head injury, metabolic imbalance, strokes, and neoplastic disease.

It is beyond the scope of this discussion to present an indepth presentation of all the types of seizures and the reader is referred to a more comprehensive reference. This presentation will be limited to tonic/clonic seizures (grand mal), absence seizures (petit mal), status epilepticus, and seizures associated with preeclampsia and eclampsia; and the drugs indicated for each type.

Tonic/clonic seizures are characterized by tonic rigidity of the extremities followed in a few seconds by a tremor. The individual then experiences the clonic phase characterized by massive jerking. In addition, the individual may experience an aura prior to the onset of a seizure. After the seizure, the patient is usually left in a fatigued state.

The absence seizure has a sudden onset and cessation lasting about 10 to 45 seconds and usually has no accompanying physical movements. The major characteristic is a momentary loss of consciousness.

Status epilepticus most often occurs as rapidly recurring tonic/clonic seizures in which the patient is unable to regain consciousness. It constitutes a medical emergency that requires medical intervention that includes the administration of medications and supportive measures.

The seizures that occur during pregnancy are of unknown origin. During pre-eclampsia the woman develops hypertension, usually with edema and proteinuria. Then she may progress to eclampsia in which she may have one or more seizures.

There are other important aspects of anticonvulsant agents important to nurses that should be included in this general discussion (Table 7–2). All agents are potentially teratogenic. Children born to mothers taking these drugs have an increased risk of having congenital malformations. Only one of the agents, phenytoin, has been associated with a specific syndrome characterized by mental retardation, nail and digital hypoplasia, facial abnormalities, and low prenatal growth. Valproic acid has been associated with an increased incidence of spina bifida. Other important aspects of patient counseling include urging the individual to wear a medical identification tag identifying the type of seizure and medication being taken. The patient should be taught factors that can precipitate seizures such as alcohol, fatigue, heat, flashing lights, and noncompliance. They should keep a seizure record and regularly make and keep appointments with the physician for drug blood level determinations and other blood or organ function tests.

Table 7–1 lists the more commonly used anticonvulsant agents.

TABLE 7-1. ANTICONVULSANT AGENTS

Generic Name	Trade Name	Use
Barbiturates		
phenobarbital[a]	Luminal	Tonic/clonic, status epilepticus
mephobarbital[a]	Mebaral	Tonic/clonic
metharbital[b]	Gemonil	Tonic/clonic
primidone[c]	Mysoline	Tonic/clonic
Benzodiazepines		
clonazepam[a]	Clonopin	Absence
diazepam[a]	Valium	Status epilepticus
Hydantoins		
phenytoin	Dilantin	Tonic/clonic, status epilepticus
ethotoin	Peganone	Tonic/clonic
mephenytoin	Mesantoin	Tonic/clonic
phenacemide	Phenurone	Tonic/clonic
Oxazolidinediones		
paramethadione	Paradione	Absence
trimethadione	Tridione	Absence
Succinimides		
ethosuximide	Zarontin	Absence
methsuximide	Celontin	Absence
phensuximide	Milontin	Absence
Miscellaneous agents		
acetazolamide	Diamox	Absence, diuretic
carbamazepine	Tegretol	Tonic/clonic, mixed seizures, trigeminal neuralgia
magnesium sulfate	—	Seizures associated with pre-eclampsia and eclampsia
valproic acid	Depakene	Absence, mixed seizures

[a] Controlled substance class CIV.
[b] Controlled substance class CIII.
[c] Not a true barbiturate, but chemically related.

BARBITURATES

Action and Fate. The exact mechanism by which the barbiturates raise seizure threshold, thus limiting the spread of seizure activity, is not known.

The barbiturates are metabolized in the liver to active and inactive products and excreted in the urine. Mephobarbital and primidone (not a true barbiturate but closely related) are metabolized to phenobarbital. Metharbital is metabolized to barbital, an active metabolite. These agents will cross the placenta.

Use. The barbiturates are effective in the prophylatic management of tonic/clonic seizures.

TABLE 7-2. GENERAL GUIDELINES FOR ANTICONVULSIVE THERAPY

1. Drug therapy is initiated with a single drug indicated for the type of epilepsy. Initially the lowest dose is given and gradually increased until seizures are controlled or toxic effects are observed.

2. If seizure control is not achieved with a single drug, a second drug is added to the regimen.

3. Once seizure control is achieved, it is important to continue to monitor the individual. Routine blood levels of the drugs and specific organ-function tests should be done and the individual instructed to record the occurrence of seizures. The individual should also be taught to avoid situations that can precipitate seizures. These include fatigue, prolonged exposure to the sun, alcohol intake, and flashing lights.

4. Anticonvulsant drugs are never abruptly discontinued. They must be gradually tapered off to prevent the occurrence of status epilepticus.

TABLE 7–3. THERAPEUTIC BLOOD LEVELS OF SOME ANTICONVULSANT AGENTS

Generic Name	Trade Name	Therapeutic Blood Level Range (mcg/ml)
phenobarbital	Luminal	10–40
mephobarbital	Mebaral	10–40[a]
primidone	Mysoline	5–10 10–40[a]
clonazepam	Clonopin	0.02–0.08
phenytoin	Dilantin	10–20
ethosuximide	Zarontin	50–100
carbamazepine	Tegretol	4–10
valproic acid	Depakene	50–100

[a] These agents are metabolized to phenobarbital and these figures reflect the phenobarbital level.

Side and Adverse Effects. Initially most individuals will experience drowsiness or sedation. In children and the elderly, these drugs may produce paradoxical excitation and hyperactive behavior. Phenobarbital infused intravenously at a rate greater than 60 mg/min may cause respiratory depression. Physiological dependence also occurs with barbiturates. Prolonged use may cause osteomalacia and folic acid deficiency.

Contraindications and Cautions. Safe use during pregnancy for barbiturates is not established. Cautious use in patients with hepatic, renal, or cardiac dysfunction.

NURSING IMPLICATIONS

- Baseline CBCs should be obtained and periodic blood tests made every 6 months.
- Warn patient of sedation that can occur.
- Blood should be monitored every 6 months for low levels of folic acid and calcium levels (Table 7–3).
- Other central nervous system (CNS) depressing substances should be avoided.
- Phenobarbital and mephobarbital are classed as CIV controlled substances. Metharbital is classed as a CIII.

BENZODIAZEPINES

Action and Fate. The exact mechanism of action of the benzodiazepines is not known. In animal studies, they apparently prevent the spread of seizure activity in the brain caused by abnormal neuronal discharges.

The benzodiazepines are excreted in the urine either as metabolites or unchanged. They can cross the placenta and appear in breast milk.

Uses. The benzodiazepines are primarily used in the management of absence seizures. Diazepam, administered intravenously, is considered to be a drug of choice in terminating status epilepticus.

Side and Adverse Effects. The benzodiazepines produce the CNS side effects common to most anticonvulsant drugs, i.e., drowsiness, ataxia, and headache. Paradoxical agitation may occur in children and the elderly. Rapid administration of diazepam IV push may cause cardiovascular collapse, therefore the administration rate should not exceed 5 mg/min. Individuals may develop both physiological and psychological dependency to benzodiazepines.

Contraindications and Cautions. These agents are contraindicated in liver disease and acute narrow angle glaucoma. Safe use during pregnancy has not been established.

NURSING IMPLICATIONS

- Baseline CBCs should be obtained and monitored every 6 months.
- Warn patient of sedation that occurs.
- Other CNS depressing substances should be avoided.
- Clonazepam and diazepam are classed as CIV controlled substances.
- IV push rate of diazepam should not exceed 5 mg/min.

HYDANTOINS

Action and Fate. The hydantoins block the sodium channels preventing the intraneuronal diffusion of sodium ions. They also reduce the influx of calcium ions. Both of these actions inhibit the development and spread of seizure activity.

The hydantoins are metabolized in the liver and excreted via bile and urine.

Uses. These agents are very effective in the management of tonic/clonic seizures. Phenytoin is also effective as an alternate for terminating status epilepticus. Its use is also indicated in the control of certain arrhythmias, specifically those caused by digitalis toxicity.

Side and Adverse Effects. Hydantoins, unlike the benzodiazepines and barbiturates, do not cause sedation. Nystagmus, ataxia, and diplopia are early dose-related side effects that require dosage reduction. Gingival hyperplasia (gum overgrowth) and hirsutism occur mostly in children. Chronic use of these drugs may cause alteration in vitamin D metabolism causing osteomalacia. They may also cause low folate levels, which result in megaloblastic anemia.

Contraindications and Cautions. All of the hydantoins should be used cautiously in hepatic or renal impairment. These agents also increase the risk of various congenital birth defects if taken during pregnancy.

NURSING IMPLICATIONS

- Baseline CBCs should be obtained and monitored every 6 months.
- Folic acid and calcium levels should also be monitored.
- Early signs of toxic levels are nystagmus, ataxia, and slurred speech.
- Shake suspension vigorously to ensure uniform distribution of drug.
- Phenytoin is *not* administered intramuscularly. The preferred route is by IV push at a rate of 50 mg/min. IV administration requires monitoring of pulse, blood pressure, and respiration. Avoid admixture with other drugs and dextrose-containing solutions. Flush line before and after administration with normal saline.
- Instruct patient on proper oral hygiene to prevent gingival hyperplasia.
- Instruct patient to avoid the use of aspirin. Aspirin will increase blood levels of phenytoin.

OXAZOLIDINEDIONES

Action and Fate. These agents elevate seizure threshold in the cortex and basal ganglia. They also reduce synaptic response to repetitive low frequency impulses.

The oxazolidinediones are metabolized in the liver to active metabolites which are excreted in the urine.

Use. This class of anticonvulsant agents is indicated in the management of absence seizures not controlled by other drugs.

Side and Adverse Effects. Drowsiness, alopecia, and hiccups occur during early treatment. A variety of visual disturbances such as photophobia, hemeralopia (day blindness), and diplopia also occur. These agents can also cause serious adverse reactions that may be fatal and that limit their usefulness. These include exfoliate dermatitis, erythema multiforme, nephropathy, hepatitis, and bone marrow depression.

Contraindications and Cautions. The use of these agents is contraindicated in individuals with severe renal or hepatic impairment and blood dyscrasias. Safe use during pregnancy has not been established. Cautious use in those with diseases of the retina and optic nerve.

NURSING IMPLICATIONS

- Initially, the administration of these medications requires close medical supervision. Liver function tests, baseline CBCs, and urinalysis should be done for baseline values and at monthly intervals for 1 year.
- Instruct patient to report any signs or symptoms that could indicate a blood dyscrasia such as onset of fever, sore throat, or unexplained bleeding.

SUCCINIMIDES

Action and Fate. These agents control seizure by the same mechanism as the oxazolidinediones. They are excreted in the urine either as metabolites or unchanged drug.

Use. All the succinimides are used to manage absence seizures. Ethosuximide is considered to be the drug of choice for this type of seizure.

Side and Adverse Effects. The most common adverse effects of these agents are related to gastrointestinal symptoms: anorexia, cramps, abdominal pain, diarrhea, nausea, and vomiting. Adverse CNS effects include drowsiness, headache, fatigue, and dizziness. Succinimides have also been associated with various blood dyscrasias, such as agranulocytosis and aplastic anemia.

Contraindications and Cautions. The use of these agents is contraindicated in those with severe liver or kidney impairment due to drug accumulation. Safe use during pregnancy has not been established.

NURSING IMPLICATIONS

- Patient should have baseline and periodic blood, renal, and hepatic function tests.
- Advise patient to avoid activities such as driving or operating machinery that requires mental alertness and motor coordination.

MISCELLANEOUS AGENTS

Acetazolamide

Action and Fate. Acetazolamide is a carbonic anhydrase inhibitor classed both as a diuretic and an anticonvulsant. Its exact mechanism of anticonvulsant activity is unknown, but it is thought to be a result of carbonic anhydrase inhibition in the CNS which retards abnormal neural discharges.

Acetazolamide is excreted unchanged in the urine. It crosses the placenta.

Use. Acetazolamide may be used in combination with other anticonvulsant agents for absence seizures. Its usefulness, however, is limited because of the tolerance to its antiseizure activity that eventually develops.

Side and Adverse Effects. Acetazolamide causes gastrointestinal side effects: anorexia, nausea, vomiting. Electrolyte disturbances can occur (e.g., hypokalemia) because of the drug's diuretic effect. Other side effects include depression, lethargy, dysuria, crystalluria, and renal colic.

Contraindications and Cautions. Acetazolamide should not be given to patients who are hypersensitive to sulfonamides. It is also contraindicated in renal or hepatic impairment, Addison's disease, electrolyte imbalances, and pregnancy. It should be used with caution in gout.

NURSING IMPLICATIONS

- Patient's potassium level should be closely monitored. Potassium supplements may be required.
- Patient should be instructed to maintain adequate fluid intake to counter diuretic effect of drug.
- Increases in blood glucose levels have been reported in diabetics, which require adjustment of diabetic medication.

Carbamazepine

Action and Fate. Carbamazepine's anticonvulsant activity involves depression of seizure propagation similar to that of phenytoin.

Metabolites and unchanged drug are excreted in the urine. Carbamazepine crosses the placenta and small amounts may appear in breast milk.

Use. Carbamazepine is indicated in the treatment of tonic/clonic seizures.

Side and Adverse Effects. Reactions that occur early in therapy but later subside include drowsiness, dizziness, ataxia, nausea, vomiting, and lightheadedness. Gastrointestinal reactions that occur include gastric distress, abdominal pain, diarrhea, constipation, and anorexia. Carbamazepine may also cause serious blood dycrasias (leukopenia, agranulocytosis, eosinophilia, leukocytosis, aplastic anemia, and thrombocytopenia).

Contraindications and Cautions. Carbamazepine is contraindicated in cardiac, renal, hepatic, or urinary tract diseases. Its use should also be avoided in patients with hypertension. Safe use during pregnancy has not been established.

NURSING IMPLICATIONS

- Complete physical evaluation and blood, hepatic, and renal function tests should be obtained prior to therapy.
- Initially, blood studies should be made weekly. After the third month, blood studies should be done on a monthly basis for 3 years.
- Instruct patient for signs and symptoms of possible blood dyscrasias such as fever, sore throat, malaise, unexplained bleeding.
- Warn patient to avoid activities that require mental alertness and physical coordination, especially during initial period.

Magnesium Sulfate

Action and Fate. When administered parenterally in sufficient quantity, magnesium sulfate depresses the CNS and blocks peripheral neuromuscular transmission.

Magnesium sulfate is excreted in the urine. It crosses the placenta easily and is found in breast milk.

Use. The primary use of magnesium sulfate as an anticonvulsant agent is to prevent and control seizures associated with severe pre-eclampsia and eclampsia in pregnant women.

Side and Adverse Effects. Adverse reactions are due to hypermagnesia. These include flushing, sweating, hypotension, depression of reflexes, circulatory collapse, and CNS depression. If not corrected, the patient can experience fatal respiratory depression.

Contraindications and Cautions. Magnesium sulfate should not be administered intravenously 2 hours before delivery. Cautious use in patients with renal impairment.

NURSING IMPLICATIONS

- Monitor patient for magnesium toxicity, profound thirst, feeling of warmth, sedation, confusion, depressed deep tendon reflexes, and muscle weakness.
- Monitor input–output ratio.
- Neonates of mothers who have received magnesium sulfate prior to delivery should be observed for magnesium toxicity and respiratory and neuromuscular depression.
- Antidote for hypermagnesemia is calcium gluconate or calcium gluceptate.

Valproic Acid

Action and Fate. The mechanism of action of valproic acid appears to be related to an increased concentration in the brain of the inhibitory neurotransmitter, gamma-aminobutyric acid (GABA).

Valproic acid is metabolized in the liver and then excreted in the urine. It crosses the placenta and is found in breast milk.

Uses. Valproic acid may be used alone or in combination with other agents in the treatment of absence seizures. It is also used with other agents in the management of certain mixed seizures.

Side and Adverse Effects. The most frequent side effects are gastrointestinal disturbances (nausea, vomiting, indigestion). Valproic acid may cause serious hepatotoxicity, which may be severe and has been responsible for a number of fatalities.

Contraindications and Cautions. Cautious use in hepatic and renal dysfunction, and angina pectoris. Safe use during pregnancy has not been established.

NURSING IMPLICATIONS

- Administer drug with meals to minimize gastric upset.
- Hepatic function should be monitored with valproic acid. Patient should be instructed to report symptoms such as rash, jaundice, light-colored stools, and vomiting.
- Warn patient of decreased mental alertness and motor coordination.

Review Questions

1–10. Matching: (Some agents have two answers.)

Agent	Seizure Type
1. _____ phenytoin	a. Tonic/clonic
2. _____ paramethadione	b. Absence
3. _____ ethosuximide	c. Status epilepticus
4. _____ acetazolamide	d. Eclampsia
5. _____ valproic acid	e. Mixed seizures
6. _____ primidone	
7. _____ diazepam	
8. _____ magnesium sulfate	
9. _____ carbamazepine	
10. _____ phenobarbital	

11. The therapeutic blood level range for phenobarbital is:
    a. 4–10 mcg/ml
    b. 10–20 mcg/ml
    c. 10–40 mcg/ml
    d. 50–75 mcg/ml

12. The therapeutic blood level range for phenytoin is:
    a. 4–10 mcg/ml
    b. 10–20 mcg/ml
    c. 10–40 mcg/ml
    d. 50–75 mcg/ml

13. Primidone is:
    a. excreted unchanged via the kidneys
    b. metabolized in the liver to two active metabolites
    c. metabolized in the liver to two inactive metabolites
    d. excreted unchanged via the bile

14. Patients whose seizures are controlled with valproic acid should have periodic _____ function tests.
    a. cardiac
    b. kidney
    c. thyroid
    d. liver

15. Signs and symptoms of hypermagnesemia include:
    a. dry mouth
    b. dilated pupils
    c. CNS depression
    d. hypertension

16. Magnesium sulfate overdose can be reversed by giving _____.

17. The nursing teaching plan for a patient taking phenytoin would include instructing the patient to:
    a. practice meticulous oral hygiene
    b. report any visual disturbances
    c. take this medication only in stressful situations
    d. rise slowly from a sitting position

18–23. Match the generic drug name found in column A with the most accurate descriptive phrase found in column B.

Column A

18. _____ valproic acid
19. _____ paramethadione
20. _____ ethosuximide
21. _____ carbamazepine
22. _____ phenytoin
23. _____ acetazolamide

Column B

a. avoid the use of aspirin with this medication
b. also used as a diuretic
c. also used for trigeminal neuralgia
d. different visual disturbances associated with this agent
e. high incidence of gastrointestinal upset
f. drug of choice for absence seizures

24. The IV push rate for diazepam should not exceed:
    a. 20 mg/min
    b. 15 mg/min
    c. 10 mg/min
    d. 5 mg/min

25. The IV push rate for phenytoin should not exceed:
    a. 100 mg/min
    b. 75 mg/min
    c. 50 mg/min
    d. 25 mg/min

=8=

Antiarthritics and Drugs for Gout

Antiarthritics

Rheumatoid arthritis is the most common of the inflammatory diseases. Before the age of 50, it occurs more frequently in women; after 50 it occurs equally in both sexes. Clinically it is characterized by inflammation of the joints and the destruction of bone and cartilage. Individuals with rheumatoid arthritis experience morning stiffness, pain associated with motion, tenderness or swelling of multiple joints (usually symmetrical), and tiredness. The formation of subcutaneous nodules also occurs.

Osteoarthritis, on the other hand, is described as a degenerative joint disease and is usually considered as an integral part of the aging process. It is not considered to be a systemic inflammatory disease, but rather a degenerative process usually confined to certain joints with some localized inflammation.

There is no cure for either disease and, for both types of arthritis, the primary goal is reduction of pain and inflammation. The initial drug of choice, both for the reduction of pain and inflammation, is aspirin. Only if the individual is not responsive or intolerant to aspirin is one of the newer nonsteroidal anti-inflammatory agents used. For resistant cases of the disease, drugs such as adrenal corticosteroids, antimalarials, immunosuppressants, gold compounds, or penicillamine may be tried. These agents are listed in Table 8–1.

NONSTEROIDAL ANTI-INFLAMMATORY AGENTS: ASPIRIN

For this group of drugs only aspirin will be discussed individually; for the other agents refer to Table 8–1.

Action and Fate. Aspirin is one of the most versatile drugs. It possesses anti-inflammatory, analgesic, antipyretic, antiplatelet actions, and has an effect on uric acid excretion (see the sixth Nursing Implication following). Its anti-inflammatory action is due to an inhibition of prostaglandin synthesis and occurs at doses of about 5 to 6 Gm/day. This is much higher than the antipyretic and analgesic action which require doses of 325 to 650 mg every 4 to 6 hours. The antiplatelet action, however, can occur with doses as low as 80 mg once a day. Aspirin is metabolized in the liver and excreted in the urine. It crosses the placenta and is found in breast milk.

Uses. In addition to its use as an anti-inflammatory agent, aspirin is used to relieve pain of low to moderate intensity such as headache, dysmenorrhea, neu-

TABLE 8–1. AGENTS USED TO REDUCE INFLAMMATION ASSOCIATED WITH ARTHRITIC CONDITIONS

Generic Name	Trade Name	Route of Administration	Dose Ranges	Adverse Effects
Nonsteroidal anti-inflammatory agents				
aspirin	Ascriptin Bufferin Cama Ecotrin Others	PO, rectally	Up to 5.4 Gm/day	Nausea, vomiting, GI distress, GI ulceration, blood loss, decreased platelet activity, aggravation of bleeding disorders, hypersensitivity reactions
diflunisal	Dolobid	PO	500 mg–1 Gm/day	GI distress, drowsiness, dizziness, confusion
fenoprofen	Nalfon	PO	1.2–2.4 Gm/day	Nausea, vomiting, GI distress, anorexia, abdominal pain, constipation
ibuprofen	Motrin Rufen	PO	1.2–2.4 Gm/day	Same as fenoprofen
indomethacin	Indocin	PO	50–200 mg/day	Nausea, GI distress, GI ulceration, blood dyscrasias, edema
meclofenamate	Meclomen	PO	200–400 mg/day	Nausea, GI distress, rash, headache, dizziness, tinnitus
naproxen	Naprosyn	PO	500–750 mg/day	GI distress, GI bleeding, abdominal pain
phenylbutazone	Butazolidin	PO	100–600 mg/day	GI distress, edema, bone dyscrasias, hypersensitivity reactions, blurred vision, bone marrow depression
piroxicam	Feldene	PO	20 mg/day	GI distress, peptic ulcer
sulindac	Clinoril	PO	300–400 mg/day	Nausea, vomiting, abdominal cramps
tolmetin	Tolectin	PO	600–1800 mg/day	Nausea, vomiting, GI distress, GI bleeding
Antimalarial agents				
chloroquine	—	PO	25 mg/day	Headache, dizziness, visual disturbances, tinnitus, anorexia, nausea, vomiting, blood dyscrasias
hydroxychloroquine	Plaquenil	PO	200–400 mg/day	Same as chloroquine
Gold compounds				
auroanofin	Ridura	PO	6 mg/day	Same as aurothioglucose
aurothioglucose	Solaganal	IM	Given at weekly intervals: Week 1: 10 mg Week 2: 25 mg Week 3 and thereafter 50 mg. If no response after a total dose of 800 mg or 1 Gm, drug should be discontinued	Stomatitis, dermatitis, blood dyscrasias, renal damage
Other agents				
azathioprine	Imuran	PO	50–100 mg/day	Blood dyscrasias, bone marrow depression
cyclophosphamide	Cytoxan	PO, IV	Use for arthritis investigation; no recommended dosage	Blood dyscrasias, bone marrow depression, hemorrhagic cystitis
penicillamine	Cuprimine Depen	PO	500–750 mg/day	Pruritis, rash, urticaria, fever, joint pain, blood dyscrasias, renal and hepatic damage

ralgia, and myalgia. The analgesia produced by a 650-mg (10-gr) tablet is equivalent to about 30 mg (1/2 gr) of codeine. Aspirin is also used to reduce fever in selected conditions and experimentally as an antiplatelet agent.

Side and Adverse Effects. Adverse reactions can be classed as hypersensitivity reactions, gastric irritation, anticoagulant action, and toxicity. Allergic reactions to aspirin include wheezing, tightness in chest, shortness of breath, urticaria, and anaphylaxis. Aspirin is highly irritating to the gastrointestinal tract and can cause nausea, vomiting, heartburn, and ulceration with occult blood. The antiplatelet action of aspirin will prolong bleeding time.

Aspirin intoxication can range from mild intoxication (salicylism) to marked toxicity. Mild intoxication causes hyperventilation, tinnitus, reversible hearing loss, dizziness, severe headache, and hypoglycemia. Marked toxicity progresses to tachycardia, pulmonary edema, hypo- or hyperglycemia, electrolyte and acid-base disturbances, central nervous system (CNS) stimulation, then CNS depression, delirium, coma, and respiratory failure.

Contraindications and Cautions. Aspirin should not be given to anyone with a known hypersensitivity to the drug or to anyone with any one of the conditions associated with the ASA triad (hayfever, nasal polyps, asthma); it should not be given to individuals with past or present history of ulcers, gastrointestinal bleeding, hemophilia, or any other bleeding disorder; or to individuals taking anticoagulants. A possible relationship between the administration of aspirin as an antipyretic and the development of Reye's syndrome in children with viral infections, has led to the recommendation that its use be avoided in children.

NURSING IMPLICATIONS

- Gastrointestinal side effects may be minimized if aspirin is given with food or milk.
- Advise individuals not to take aspirin if alcohol has been consumed, in order to avoid added irritation to the gastrointestinal system.
- Aspirin should not be administered to any individual with bleeding disorders or during pregnancy and postpartum because of its antiplatelet effect.
- Assess patients for ASA triad before administering aspirin.
- Avoid use of aspirin in children without consulting a physician.
- One to 2 Gm of aspirin daily decreases uric acid excretion; 5 Gm or more daily increases uric acid excretion. These alterations in uric acid excretion indicate that the use of aspirin should be avoided in individuals with gout.
- Aspirin should be avoided with the following drugs: anticoagulants, corticosteroids, indomethacin, methotrexate, oral hypoglycemic agents, phenytoin, uricosuric agents, and phenylbutazone.

OTHER ANTI-INFLAMMATORY AGENTS

The action of the remaining nonsteroidal anti-inflammatory agents is similar to aspirin. For most, use is limited to reducing inflammation associated with arthritic conditions. Exceptions are ibuprofen, which may be used as an analgesic for headache or dysmenorrhea and naproxen, which may be used for dysmenorrhea.

All these agents are associated with severe gastrointestinal irritation, which limits their use in many cases. There is a high incidence of blood dyscrasias with indomethacin, phenylbutazone, and meclofenamate.

Penicillamine

Penicillamine is a byproduct of penicillin hydrolysis that lacks any antibacterial activity. Its primary indication is as a chelating agent for heavy metal poisoning.

Its pharmacological action in rheumatoid arthritis is not known. The most common adverse effects are skin rashes and gastrointestinal upsets. More serious adverse effects are renal damage and bone marrow depression. Patients who have a history of allergic reactions to penicillin should avoid taking penicillamine.

Adrenal Corticosteroids

The adrenal corticosteroids are used when more conventional treatment has failed. Orally, prednisone is the corticosteroid most frequently employed. Long-acting parenteral preparations may be injected directly into the affected joint (intra-articularly). A more detailed discussion of the adrenal corticosteroids is given in Chapter 11.

Immunosuppressive Agents

Two agents fall into this category, azathioprine and cyclophosphamide. These two agents are used as a last resort in cases of severe, progressive rheumatoid arthritis.

Both agents can cause nausea, vomiting, and bone marrow depression. Additional adverse effects of cyclophosphamide are hemorrhagic cystitis and the future development of malignancies. For both agents the patient should be closely monitored and complete blood counts performed at regular intervals.

Nursing Implications for Penicillamine, Adrenal Corticosteroids, and Immunosuppressive Agents

- Give these medications with food and milk to minimize gastrointestinal distress.
- Patients with aspirin hypersensitivity should avoid these agents also.
- Blood tests should be performed twice a year for patients taking indomethacin, phenylbutazone, or meclofenamate.
- Indomethocin should be used cautiously in patients with cardiovascular disorders because of the edema it may cause.

Drugs for Gout

Gout is a syndrome characterized by an elevated uric acid blood level (hyperuricemia) and by episodes of severe, acute attacks of arthritis. If left untreated the disease progresses through four stages: (1) asymptomatic hyperuricemia, (2) acute gouty arthritis, (3) interval period, and (4) chronic tophaceous gout. Tophaceous gout is characterized by urate deposits in the cartilage of the ear pinna, big toe, bursae, tendons, skin, and kidneys. If diagnosed and treated early, the progress of the disease can be stopped before it progresses to the fourth stage.

Hyperuricemia occurs as a result of either (1) an inborn error of metabolism that causes an overproduction of uric acid (these individuals are classed as overproducers) or (2) a decreased ability of the kidneys to secrete uric acid (these individuals are classed as undersecretors). Hyperuricemia may also develop as a result of a disease or drug treatment that is associated with an increase in cell destruction, which in turn results in an increased breakdown of nucleic acid of which uric acid is a byproduct.

TABLE 8–2. DRUGS USED SPECIFICALLY TO TREAT GOUT

Generic Name	Trade Name	Route of Administration	Dose Ranges	Adverse Effects
allopurinol	Lopurin Zyloprim	PO	200–300 mg/day, maximum dose 800 mg/day	Rash, nausea, vomiting, diarrhea, blood dyscrasias
colchicine	—	PO, IV	For acute gouty attack—PO: 0.5 or 0.6 mg/hr or 1 or 1.2 mg initially, followed by 0.5 or 0.6 mg/2 hr until pain subsides or diarrhea occurs IV: 1 or 2 mg initially followed by 0.5 mg q12h or q24h until pain subsides For prophylaxis—PO: 0.5 or 1.5 mg/day	Nausea, vomiting, diarrhea, blood dyscrasias, tissue necrosis if IV infusion extravasates
probenecid	Benemid	PO	0.5–2 Gm/day	Headache, GI distress, anemia, sore gums, hypersensitivity reactions
sulfinpyrazone	Anturane	PO	200–400 mg/day	GI distress, rash

The symptoms of an acute gouty attack result from a systemic inflammatory reaction to the formation of urate crystals in synovial fluids. The aim of therapy is twofold: (1) the termination of the inflammatory process associated with an acute attack and (2) the reduction of uric acid levels in the blood in order to promote the resolution of urate deposits and to prevent further formation of uric acid deposits and acute gouty attacks.

Treatment of an acute gouty attack is usually with colchicine and one of the nonsteroidal anti-inflammatory agents. Drug selection for the long-term management of gout depends on whether the patient is an overproducer or undersecretor (Table 8–2). For an overproducer the drug usually used is allopurinol; for an undersecretor, probenecid.

GOUT SUPPRESSANT TREATMENT: COLCHICINE

Action and Fate. Colchicine interferes with the formation of microtubules in certain cells that are mobile, thus interfering with their movement. In the case of gout, the therapeutic action of colchicine is thought to inhibit the migration of leukocytes and the phagocytosis that occurs in joints that contain urate crystals. This action of the drug reduces the pain and inflammation associated with gout.

The drug is partially metabolized in the liver. Metabolites and active drugs are primarily excreted in the feces.

Uses. Colchicine is the drug of choice for treating an acute attack of gouty arthritis. It may also be used prophylactically to prevent recurrent attacks. It can be used alone or in combination with one of the other antigout medications used to reduce uric acid blood levels.

Side and Adverse Effects. Colchicine causes a variety of gastrointestinal side effects including nausea, vomiting, and diarrhea. These effects are early signs of toxicity. The diarrhea that occurs may require treatment if severe. The drug can also cause bone marrow depression (leukopenia, thrombocytopenia, agranulocytosis, and aplastic anemia). Extravasation of colchicine during IV administration can cause tissue necrosis.

Contraindications and Cautions. The parenteral form of colchicine is administered IV only. It should not be used in individuals with blood dyscrasias, gastrointestinal, renal, hepatic, or cardiac disease. Cautious use in the elderly.

NURSING IMPLICATIONS

- Baseline and periodic blood counts should be done.
- When given orally the drug may be administered with food or milk to minimize gastrointestinal upset.
- Drugs that mask diarrhea, an early sign of toxicity, should not be administered to patients while on medication. However, antidiarrheals may be given to treat diarrhea once colchicine has been discontinued.
- Encourage increased fluid intake.
- Advise patients to report symptoms of bone marrow depression (sore mouth, bleeding, fever, malaise, and sore throat).

URICOSURIC AGENTS

Probenecid

Action and Fate. Probenecid is a sulfonamide derivative that inhibits renal tubular reabsorption of uric acid (Fig. 8–1), promoting the excretion and reducing blood levels of uric acid. Probenecid also prevents the formation of new urate deposits and causes gradual reduction of old deposits.

Probenecid is metabolized by the liver and excreted as metabolites and active drug in the urine. It crosses the placenta.

Uses. Used to promote excretion of uric acid in chronic gouty arthritis and tophaceous gout. It is also used to block the excretion of penicillin-type antibiotics in order to prolong therapeutic concentrations in the body.

Side and Adverse Effects. Most frequently, patients will experience headache, nausea, vomiting, and anorexia. Nephrotic syndrome, hepatic necrosis, and aplastic anemia may also occur.

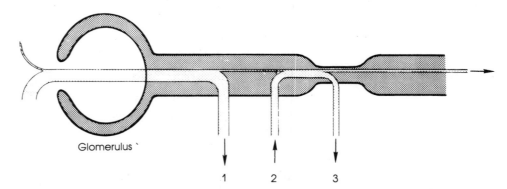

Glomerulus

1   2   3

Figure 8–1. All but the protein-bound urate is filtered into the urine at the glomerulus. At site 1, in the proximal tubule practically all of the uric acid is reabsorbed into the bloodstream. The uricosuric agents—probenecid, sulfinpyrazone, and large doses of aspirin—act at this site to inhibit uric acid reabsorption. At site 2, also in the proximal tubule, about half of the uric acid reabsorbed is excreted back into urine. Here low or usual doses of aspirin decrease the amount of uric acid that is excreted into the urine. At site 3, about 80 percent of the excreted uric acid is reabsorbed. (*Adapted from Meyers FH, Jawetz E, Goldfien A [eds]: Review of Medical Pharmacology, ed 7. Los Altos, Calif, Lange Medical Publications, 1980, with permission.*)

Contraindications and Cautions. Probenecid should not be used in individuals with uric acid kidney stones, during or within 2 to 3 weeks of an acute gouty attack; in individuals who are overexcretors of uric acid (over 1000 mg/day); in individuals with a kidney creatinine clearance of less than 50 mg/min; or in individuals with hyperuricemia secondary to cancer chemotherapy. Cautious use in those with history of peptic ulcer disease.

NURSING IMPLICATIONS

- Gastrointestinal side effects can be minimized if the medication is taken with food or milk.
- Increased water intake to 3000 ml/day is recommended in order to decrease the possibility of the formation of renal calculi (stones) due to the increased concentration of uric acid excreted.
- Oral sodium bicarbonate may be prescribed to alkalinize the urine as another means of preventing the formation of renal calculi.
- Agents that tend to acidify the urine such as vitamin C or cranberry juice should be avoided since an acidic urine pH will promote the formation of renal calculi.

Sulfinpyrazone

Action and Fate. Like probenicid, sulfinpyrazone promotes the excretion of uric acid by inhibiting renal tubular reabsorption. It also decreases platelet adhesiveness.

Sulfinpyrazone is metabolized in the liver to active and inactive metabolites.

Uses. Sulfinpyrazone is used for the management of chronic gouty arthritis and tophaceous gout. It may also be used for prophylactic treatment of myocardial infarction since it inhibits platelet aggregation and may decrease the formation of blood clots in coronary vessels.

Side and Adverse Effects. Sulfinpyrazone commonly causes gastrointestinal disturbances. It may also cause inner ear disturbances, edema, and convulsions.

Contraindications and Cautions. Sulfinpyrazone should not be used in individuals with active peptic ulcer, or with a kidney creatinine clearance less than 50 mg/min. It is not used for treatment of hyperuricemia secondary to cancer chemotherapy.

NURSING IMPLICATIONS

- Administer these drugs with food or milk to minimize gastrointestinal side effects.
- Baseline blood counts and renal function tests should be done prior to treatment and periodically after treatment is initiated.
- Advise patient to increase fluid intake to 3000 ml/day.
- Sulfinpyrazone initially will increase frequency of acute gouty attacks.
- Advise patient to avoid the use of aspirin since it can exacerbate gout.
- Sulfinpyrazone may enhance the effects of anticoagulants and it may enhance the hypoglycemic effects of the oral hypoglycemia agents.

XANTHINE OXIDASE INHIBITOR: ALLOPURINOL

Action and Fate. Allopurinol is not classed as an uricosuric agent like probenecid and sulfinpyrazone; it acts to inhibit the action of the enzyme xanthine oxidase.

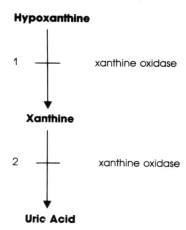

Figure 8–2. Sites 1 and 2 are the steps in the breakdown of hypoxanthine that are blocked by allopurinol and thus inhibit the formation of uric acid.

This enzyme converts hypoxanthine to xanthine and xanthine to uric acid (Fig. 8–2). Allopurinol, thus, lowers the uric acid level both in the blood and the urine.

Uses. Allopurinol is used to reduce elevated uric acid blood levels in individuals who are diagnosed as overproducers and who have severe tophaceous gout with renal insufficiency or uric acid renal calculi. It is also used prophylactically for secondary hyperuricemia resulting from cancer chemotherapy.

Side and Adverse Effects. Allopurinol can cause a number of dermatologic effects including pruritic maculopapular rash, exfoliate, urticarial, and purpural dermatitis. It also causes gastrointestinal upsets and blood dyscrasias.

Contraindications and Cautions. Allopurinol should not be used in those individuals with a known sensitivity to the drug. It should not be used as an initial treatment for an acute gouty attack. The appearance of a skin rash indicates that therapy with allopurinol should be discontinued. Safe use during pregnancy or while nursing has not been established. Cautious use is indicated in those individuals with impaired renal or hepatic function, history of peptic ulcer, or lower gastrointestinal tract disease.

NURSING IMPLICATIONS

- Medication may be administered with food or milk.
- Instruct patient to promptly report the appearance of a rash, which would signal a toxic reaction.
- Baseline blood counts and liver and kidney function tests should be done and repeated periodically.
- Acute gouty attacks usually occur during first 6 weeks of therapy and colchicine may be prescribed concurrently.
- Advise patient to maintain a fluid intake of 3000 ml/day.
- Allopurinol enhances the toxicity of the antineoplastic agent mercaptopurine and increases the risk of rash with ampicillin.
- Advise patient not to use aspirin as an analgesic since it can exacerbate gout.

Review Questions

1. It is believed that rheumatoid arthritis is an autoimmune disease. Sometimes an immunosuppressive agent such as cyclophosphamide is given. Which one

of the following symptoms would indicate an adverse effect of this type of drug?
a. hearing loss
b. peripheral neuritis
c. congestive heart failure
d. fever

2. Patients taking phenylbutazone should promptly report which of the following symptoms?
a. weight loss
b. sore throat
c. jaundice
d. diarrhea

3. Phenylbutazone should be used cautiously if a patient has:
a. glaucoma
b. diabetes
c. congestive heart failure
d. grand mal seizures

4. Which one of the following is used to help alleviate pain associated with dysmenorrhea?
a. indomethacin
b. phenylbutazone
c. ibuprofen
d. colchicine

5. Which one of the following medications would mask an important warning sign that would indicate that an excessive dose of colchicine was being taken?
a. aspirin
b. penicillin VK
c. Lomotil
d. acetaminophen

6. A patient who is a uric acid undersecretor is prescribed probenecid. The patient should be instructed to:
a. drink plenty of cranberry juice
b. avoid milk products
c. avoid the use of stool softeners
d. maintain a fluid intake of 3000 to 4000 ml per day

7. Allopurinol is given to those patients who are considered to be overproducers of uric acid. The doctor orders 100 mg twice a day. You would instruct the patient to notify the doctor if:
a. fever develops
b. edema develops
c. a rash appears
d. blurred vision occurs

8–19. Matching:

Generic Name	**Trade Name**
8. _____ibuprofen	a. Indocin
9. _____sulindac	b. Imuran
10. _____auroanofin	c. Cuprimine, Depen
11. _____allopurinol	d. Ridura
12. _____indomethacin	e. Motrin, Rufen
13. _____naproxen	f. Clinoril
14. _____sulfinpyrazone	g. Feldene

15. _____ probenicid
16. _____ phenylbutazone
17. _____ piroxicam
18. _____ azathioprine
19. _____ penicillamine

h. Anturane
i. Lopurin, Zyloprim
j. Benemid
k. Butazolidin
l. Naprosyn

9

Opioids and Nonopioid Analgesics

This section presents a review of opiates, semisynthetic and synthetic opioid derivatives, opioid antagonists, and nonopioid analgesics (Tables 9–1 and 9–2). The nonopioid agents have already been discussed in Chapter 8, under anti-arthritic agents and will not be repeated here. Only one nonopioid analgesic, the para-aminophenol derivative acetaminophen, will be presented in this section.

OPIATES AND OPIOIDS

Opium, the name given to the crude alkaloid extract, is obtained from the latex produced by the unripened seed capsule of the poppy plant, *Papaver somniferum.* Many different alkaloids are contained in this crude preparation, but only four have medical application; these are morphine, codeine, papaverine, and noscapine. Table 9–3 gives the uses and percent of each.

The physiological and psychological effects of opium were known to ancient civilizations as early as 4000 BC. Through the years, easy accessibility of opium and indiscriminate use of its major component, morphine, led to abuse and misuse of these agents. This resulted in many individuals becoming addicted. Recognition of this undesirable addiction liability has stimulated the development of analgesics that would retain the effective analgesia property but would be devoid of the addicting potential found in the opiate analgesics. These agents are classed as agonist/antagonists. Also, in an effort to prevent further abuse and misuse of these agents and agents with similar addicting potential, legislation both at the federal and state levels was enacted to control the manufacture, sale, and distribution of these substances. For this reason, these agents are known as controlled substances. (See Chapter 1 for a discussion of the legal definition of the various classes of controlled substances.)

Action and Fate. The opiates and their derivatives exert their pharmacological action by interacting with receptors located in the limbic system, the central part of the thalamus of the brain, the spinal cord, and the intestines. The analgesic action is thought to be due to either elevation of pain threshold, interference with pain conduction, altered pain perception, or a combination of these effects. Other important pharmacological effects include sedation, euphoria, drowsiness, lethargy, apathy, and mental confusion. They inhibit the cough center, stimulate the chemoreceptor trigger zone, and depress the respiratory center in the brain. They also cause hypotension and tachycardia, inhibition of parastalsis, spasm of the sphincter of Oddi, urinary retention, and pupil constriction. Tolerance can develop to most of these effects, except the effects of the gastrointestinal tract, the eye, and the chemoreceptor trigger zone.

The opiates are metabolized in the liver. In some cases a small amount of

TABLE 9–1. OPIATES AND RELATED OPIOIDS AND ANTAGONISTS

Generic Name	Trade Name	Use	Controlled Substance Class
codeine	—	Analgesia, antitussive	CII
fentanyl	Sublimaze	Preanesthesia, postoperative analgesia	CII
hydromorphone	Dilaudid	Analgesia	CII
levorphanol	Levo-Dromoran	Analgesia, preanesthesia	CII
meperidine	Demerol	Analgesia, preanesthesia, analgesia during labor and delivery	CII
methadone	Dolophine	Analgesia, substitute for heroin addiction	CII
morphine	—	Analgesia, preanesthesia	CII
opium alkaloids	Pantopon	Analgesia, preanesthesia	CII
oxycodone	in Percocet, Percodan, Tylox	Analgesia	CII
oxymorphone	Numorphan	Analgesia	CII
propoxyphene	Darvon	Analgesia	CIV

unchanged drug is also excreted via the kidneys. These agents cross the placenta and are found in breast milk.

Uses. The opiates and their derivatives are indicated for the relief of moderate to severe acute pain (Table 9–4). Selected ones are often used as preoperative medication in combination with other agents (e.g., atropine, promethazine) or alone to decrease anxiety and facilitate induction. Other selected agents are used as cough suppressants or as antidiarrheals. Morphine is used to relieve the dyspnea and pulmonary edema associated with left ventricular failure and for the pain caused by a myocardial infarct. Meperidine may be used for obstetric analgesia (Table 9–5).

Side and Adverse Effects. The opiates and related agents cause a number of undesirable effects that limit their usefulness. Depression of the central nervous system leads to drowsiness, sedation, and to decreased rate of respiration. They cause constipation, nausea, and vomiting; suppress the cough center; contract the pupils of the eyes; increase intracranial pressure; and cause a drop in blood pressure. Opiates are also associated with a histamine release that results in a rash or pruritis.

Contraindications and Cautions. Conditions that contraindicate the use of opioids include convulsive disorders, head injury, asthma and any other respiratory disease, prostatic hypertrophy, and severe kidney and liver insufficiency.

TABLE 9–2. MIXED AGONISTS–ANTAGONISTS AND OPIOID ANTAGONISTS

Generic Name	Trade Name	Use	Controlled Substance Class
Mixed agonists–antagonists			
butorphanol	Stadol	Analgesia	—
nalbuphine	Nubain	Analgesia	—
pentazocine	Talwin	Analgesia, preanesthesia	CIV
Antagonists			
naloxone	Narcan	Reversal of opiate depression due to overdose	—

TABLE 9–3. MEDICALLY USEFUL ALKALOIDS FOUND IN THE CRUDE OPIUM EXTRACT

Natural Alkaloid	Percent Found in Opium	Major Use
morphine	12	Analgesia
codeine	0.5	Analgesia, antitussive
papaverine	1	Smooth muscle relaxant
noscapine	6	Antitussive

Since most opiates and their derivatives have addicting liability, it is recommended that the smallest effective dose be used for the minimum time.

NURSING IMPLICATIONS

- It is important for the nurse to evaluate patient's need for PRN pain medication.
- Ensure that physician's order is still valid prior to administering a dose. Know the institution's stop date policy concerning controlled substances.
- It is important to assess patient's vital signs regularly. Before giving a dose, note respiratory rate, blood pressure, state of pupils, and consciousness level of patient. If patient has a respiratory rate below 12, pupils are constricted, or if in a coma, notify the physician. These signs are known as the opioid triad.
- Be prepared with supportive measures for an overdose. Have naloxone and resuscitation equipment available for use in case of an overdose per physician order.
- Encourage postoperative patients to cough and deep breathe.
- Monitor bowel movements and input–output ratio.
- After administering the medication, warn patient not to change position suddenly or ambulate without help. Side rails should be up.

OPIOID ANTAGONIST: NALOXONE

Action and Fate. Naloxone is a pure narcotic antagonist; it essentially has no intrinsic analgesic property.

The drug is rapidly metabolized by the liver and excreted via the kidneys. Naloxone does cross the placenta.

TABLE 9–4. OPIATES AND OPIOIDS LISTED ACCORDING TO RELATIVE POTENCY

Generic Name	Trade Name
Most potent	
morphine	—
hydromorphone	Dilaudid
levorphanol	Levo-Dromoran
methadone	Dolophine
oxymorphone	Numorphan
Intermediate potency	
alphaphrodine	Nisentil
butorphanol	Stadol
meperidine	Demerol
nalbuphine	Nubain
oxycodone	Percocet-5,[a] Percodan,[b] Tylox[a]
pentazocine	Talwin
Least potent	
codeine	—
dihydrocodeine	Drocode, Paracodin

[a] Combined with acetaminophen in Percocet-5 and Tylox.
[b] Combined with aspirin in Percodan.

TABLE 9–5. PHENYLPIPERIDINES: MEPERIDINE AND RELATED SYNTHETIC OPIOIDS

Generic Name	Trade Name	Controlled Substance Class
meperidine	Demerol	CII
alphaprodine	Nisentil	CII
anileridine	Leritine	CII
diphenoxylate	Lomotil[a]	CIV
loperamide	Imodium	—

[a] Combined with atropine sulfate in Lomotil.

Uses. It is used to reverse the effects of an overdose of an opiate or opioid derivative. It is also used to diagnose an overdose suspected to be caused by an opiate. It is not effective in reversing an overdose caused by a nonopioid agent.

Side and Adverse Effects. Used as recommended, naloxone is relatively free of adverse effects. An excessive dose of naloxone can cause reversal of analgesia, increased blood pressure, tremors, drowsiness, and elevated partial thromboplastin time. A too-rapid reversal of overdose can cause nausea, vomiting, sweating, and tachycardia.

Contraindications and Cautions. Naloxone should not be used in those individuals with known hypersensitivity reactions to the drug or respiratory depression due to a nonopioid drug. Use of the drug in known or suspected narcotic-dependent persons can precipitate withdrawal symptoms.

NURSING IMPLICATIONS

- Monitor patient's vital signs. In some, respirations may increase to a higher level after administration.
- Duration of opioid may exceed that of naloxone. Repeated doses of naloxone may be needed.
- Withdrawal symptoms can be induced by the administration of naloxone in individuals addicted to opiates.

NONOPIOID ANALGESIC: ACETAMINOPHEN

For discussion of aspirin see Chapter 8.

Action and Fate. Acetaminophen has analgesic and antipyretic actions. It does not have an anti-inflammatory effect. It reduces fever by direct action on the hypothalamic heat regulatory center, which causes peripheral vasodilatation and heat dissipation. Analgesia is produced by raising pain threshold by an unknown mechanism.

Acetaminophen is metabolized by the liver. Only 2 to 4 percent is excreted unchanged. Acetaminophen does cross the placenta.

Uses. Acetaminophen is used to relieve mild to moderate pain and for reduction of fever.

Side and Adverse Effects. Acetaminophen is well tolerated at recommended doses. Chronic ingestion can cause blood dyscrasias, hepatic and renal damage. Acute poisoning causes anorexia, nausea, vomiting, hepatoxicity, hepatic coma, and renal failure.

Contraindications and Cautions. Repeated administration of acetaminophen is contraindicated in patients with anemia or hepatic, renal, cardiac, or pulmonary disease. Cautious use in individuals with alcoholism or malnutrition.

NURSING IMPLICATIONS

- It is important to caution the patient to follow recommended doses and dosing frequency. Exceeding recommended doses can cause liver damage and other serious toxic effects.
- Individuals with poor nutrition or history of alcohol abuse are more prone to hepatic toxicity even at normal doses.

Review Questions

Give three sites where opiate receptors are located.

1. _____

2. _____

3. _____

4. Tolerance develops to most opiate side effects except:
   a. miosis
   b. respiratory depression
   c. analgesia
   d. sedation

5. The drug used to relieve pain associated with myocardial infarct is:
   a. Percodan
   b. codeine
   c. morphine
   d. methadone

6. For analgesia during labor and delivery, which one of the following opiates is recommended?
   a. Dilaudid
   b. Demerol
   c. Levo-Dromoran
   d. Sublimaze

Give three parameters that you should assess prior to administering an opiate (opioid triad).

7. _____

8. _____

9. _____

10. An individual addicted to opioids would not show withdrawal symptoms if given:
    a. Narcan
    b. Stadol
    c. Dilaudid
    d. Nubain

11. The dose of opiates should be decreased in case of:
    a. renal impairment
    b. decreased liver function
    c. cardiovascular disease
    d. Addison's disease

12. Prolonged use of acetaminophen at doses exceeding the recommended amount will lead to:
    a. liver damage
    b. brain damage
    c. retinopathy
    d. severe anemia

13–24. Matching:

Agent	**Controlled Substance Class**
13. _____ codeine	a. schedule II
14. _____ Demerol	b. schedule III
15. _____ Dolophine	c. schedule IV
16. _____ Darvon	d. schedule V
17. _____ Narcan	e. not a controlled substance
18. _____ Talwin	
19. _____ Percodan	
20. _____ morphine	
21. _____ methadone	
22. _____ Sublimaze	
23. _____ Stadol	
24. _____ Nubain	

25–30. Matching:

Agent	**Relative Potency**
25. _____ codeine	a. most potent
26. _____ Stadol	b. intermediate potency
27. _____ Demerol	c. least potent
28. _____ pentazocine	
29. _____ methadone	
30. _____ morphine	

Give two advantages of acetaminophen over aspirin.

31. _____

32. _____

33. Clinical uses of opiates and derivatives include the treatment of:
    a. severe pain
    b. cough
    c. diarrhea
    d. all of the above

Agents Used for Cardiovascular Conditions

Cardiac Glycosides

The therapeutic goal in the treatment of congestive heart failure (CHF) is to strengthen the force of contraction of the myocardium thus improving cardiac output. CHF is a condition in which the heart is no longer able to pump a sufficient amount of oxygenated blood to meet the metabolic demands of the body. A number of the clinical signs and symptoms of this condition are due to the various compensatory mechanisms used by the body in order to improve cardiac output (Fig. 10–1). Administration of a cardiac glycoside is an integral part of the treatment regimen which also includes rest, restricted salt intake, and diuretics.

Cardiac glycosides are also referred to as digitalis or digitalis preparations. This is a term used to refer to the cardiac glycosides as a group. The therapeutic effects of these agents have been known since the 1700s. They are natural products derived mainly from two species of foxglove plant, *Digitalis purpurea* and *Digitalis lavata*. There are still several different glycosides available; however, only two agents, digoxin and digitoxin, will be presented in this unit. A comparison of the two agents is given in Table 10–1.

Individuals receiving a cardiac glycoside require close observation. Toxic levels of the drugs can easily occur since the margin between the therapeutic blood levels and toxic blood levels is very narrow.

Action and Fate. Cardiac glycosides share a common effect on the myocardium. The exact mechanism by which they are able to strengthen the force of myocardial contraction is not known.

Apparently cardiac glycosides inhibit the Na^+, K^+ activated enzyme, ATPase. This action reduces the amount of energy available to the sodium pump and causes an increase of the intracellular concentration of Na^+. In turn, an increased intracellular concentration of Na^+ increases the intracellular concentration of Ca^{++}. As a result of this, the force of myocardial contraction is increased (a positive inotropic effect). Cardiac glycosides, therefore, increase stroke volume and cardiac output; they reduce residual diastolic volume and heart size. They improve systemic and pulmonary circulation and reduce venous blood pressure. These improvements in blood circulation also improve blood delivery to the kidneys. Therefore, cardiac glycosides initially cause an increase in urine

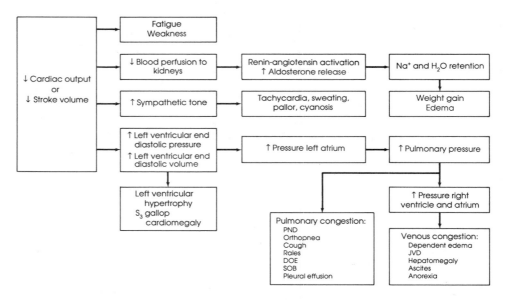

Figure 10–1. Signs and symptoms and compensatory mechanisms of congestive heart failure. (Abbreviations: PND, paroxysmal nocturnal dyspnea; DOE, dyspnea on exertion; SOB, shortness of breath; JVD, jugular venous distention.)

production even though they have no diuretic properties. Other cardiac effects attributed to cardiac glycosides are a slowing of the heart rate (a negative chronotropic effect) by direct action on the myocardium and by increasing vagal tone to the heart, and a depression of impulse formation at the sinus (SA) node and bundle tissue (a negative dromotropic effect) lengthening the refractory period.

Digitoxin is primarily metabolized in the liver and excreted via the kidneys as inactive metabolites. Digoxin is primarily excreted unchanged by the kidneys.

Uses. The cardiac glycosides are used in the treatment of heart failure. They are also used in the management of supraventricular tachycardia arrhythmias (see following section on antiarrhythmia agents).

Side and Adverse Effects. Cardiac glycosides can produce a number of undesirable effects which occur frequently because of the narrow therapeutic index of these agents. Anorexia, nausea, vomiting, and bradycardia (heart rate below 60) are frequently initial signs of toxic blood levels. In addition, the cardiac glycosides can cause fatigue, mental depression, lethargy, headache, confusion, and nightmares. Cardiac glycosides can precipitate any type of arrhythmia, with the formation of ectopic beats being the most common. These agents also can cause all grades of impaired myocardial conduction. Other side effects include disturbed vision, altered color perception, hazy vision, and seeing flickering dots and halos around objects.

TABLE 10–1. A COMPARISON OF TWO DIGITALIS PREPARATIONS: DIGOXIN AND DIGITOXIN

Generic Name	Trade Name	% Absorbed After Oral Administration	Onset of Action After Oral Administration (min)	Half-life ($t_{1/2}$)	Metabolism and Route of Excretion
digoxin	Lanoxin	75[a]	15–30	36 hr	Not metabolized, mainly excreted unchanged by the kidneys
digitoxin	Crystodigin Purodigin	95	25–120	5 days	Metabolized in the liver before being excreted

[a] Absorption varies according to manufacturer.

Contraindications and Cautions. Use of cardiac glycosides is contraindicated in those individuals with a known sensitivity to these agents and in those with ventricular fibrillation or tachycardia unless they are due to CHF. Digoxin should be used cautiously in those with impaired kidney function; digitoxin, in those with impaired liver damage. Both should be used with caution in individuals with incomplete heart block.

NURSING IMPLICATIONS

The nursing implications given focus specifically on digoxin since it is the most frequently used cardiac glycoside.

- Baseline potassium levels must be obtained prior to the initiation of treatment with digoxin and twice a year thereafter.
- If potassium level is below 3.5 mEq, hold medication and contact physician. Hypokalemia while the individual is taking digoxin enhances the formation of arrhythmias.
- Obtain apical pulse prior to administering digoxin. In adults, if the rate is below 60 or above 110, hold medication and contact physician. In children, hold medication and contact physician if rate is less than 70.
- Teach patient to take apical pulse.
- Digoxin levels should be obtained twice a year. Therapeutic range is usually 0.8 to 2.0 ng/ml, toxic level is above 2 ng/ml.
- In order to obtain therapeutic blood levels of digoxin within 24 hours for those with severe heart failure, the individual is given a loading dose or digitalizing dose. The dose is calculated on the patient's body weight in kilograms and kidney function. For an individual with normal kidney function, the dose is 0.01 to 0.02 mg/kg of body weight given in three divided doses. Drug levels are done after each dose in order to prevent an overdose. Once the patient is digitalized, a maintenance dose is given once a day to replace the amount that is excreted. For individuals with reduced kidney function, dosage reduction is calculated.
- Quinidine and calcium channel blockers interfere with the excretion of digoxin and increase risk of toxicity.
- Doses are not equivalent when changes are made in dosage form. Oral tablets deliver less systemically than equivalent amounts given intravenously or in elixir form.
- DO NOT INJECT DIGOXIN IM; this causes intense pain and absorption is erratic.
- The bioavailability of different brands of digoxin tablets varies, therefore generic substitution is not permitted.
- Avoid medications that cause fluid retention, alter heart rate, or cause cardiac damage (Table 10–2).

TABLE 10–2. DRUGS THAT CAN PRECIPITATE OR EXACERBATE CONGESTIVE HEART FAILURE

Agent or Class	Effect
Androgens and estrogens	Cause fluid retention
Glucocorticosteroids	Agents with mineralocorticoid properties can cause sodium retention
phenylbutazone	Causes fluid retention
Beta blockers	Slow heart beat
Medications high in sodium content (antacids and antibiotics)	Fluid retention
doxorubicin	Cardiotoxic agent

Antiarrhythmia Agents

The treatment of cardiac arrhythmias is extremely complex. Both the method of treatment and selection of medication depend on (1) the type of arrhythmia, (2) its location, (3) its seriousness, and (4) the patient's overall condition. The most common treatment of arrhythmias is with drugs; however, there are situations that require the placement of a mechanical pacemaker or the use of DC cardioversion in order to reinstate a normal sinus rhythm.

In order to relate the action of antiarrhythmia agents, a brief review of basic electrophysiology of cardiac tissue will be given prior to discussing the drugs.

BASIC CARDIAC ELECTROPHYSIOLOGY

In the heart there is a specialized system of muscle tissue that can initiate and transmit electrical impulses to the atria and ventricles. This results in a coordinated pumping action that delivers in a very efficient way oxygenated blood to the various parts of the body.

Those cells in the heart that are able to depolarize spontaneously, initiating electrical impulses that give rise to a normal heart beat, are said to possess a characteristic known as automaticity. The major location of these specialized cells is the SA node, which is also known as the pacemaker. In addition, there are other or secondary sites of pacemaker cells located at the atrioventricular (AV) node and the His-Purkinje system. These secondary sites will begin to depolarize spontaneously if for some reason the SA node is not generating impulses. When the secondary sites do begin to function they are known as ectopic pacemakers.

The normal course of events, however, is for an electrical impulse to be generated at the SA node, travel through the atria and cause their contraction.

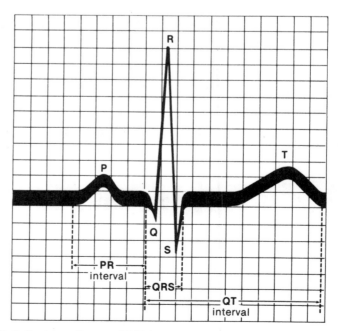

Figure 10–2. Electrocardiogram (ECG) tracing showing the patterns typical of normal heart function. *(From Gomella LG (ed): Clinician's Pocket Reference, 5th ed. East Norwalk, Conn, Appleton & Lange, 1986, with permission.)*

This atrial depolarization is represented on the electrocardiogram (ECG) as the P wave (Fig. 10–2). The impulse then travels to the AV node, the only pathway between the atria and ventricles. The AV node should be thought of as a control center since it regulates the number of impulses that reach the ventricles. The AV node can also regulate ventricular rate if the pacemaker cells begin to depolarize too quickly, i.e., generating impulses too quickly.

After the electrical impulse has passed the AV node, it enters the bundle of His, a type of specialized conducting tissue. The bundle of His then divides into right and left branches, one for each ventricle. Eventually each branch further subdivides into smaller branches known as Purkinje fibers. The QRS complex on the ECG represents ventricular depolarization, while the T wave corresponds to ventricular repolarization.

Membrane Potentials

All cardiac cells inherently possess an electrical potential that keeps the intracellular part of cardiac cells electrically negative relative to the outer part (Fig. 10–3). At rest the cell membrane potential will usually register at -70 or -90 MV. At this time, the cell membrane is more permeable to K^+, allowing this ion to readily diffuse out of the cell, and less permeable to Na^+, Cl^-, and Ca^{++}. The loss of K^+ from the inside of the cell and the accumulation of Na^+ and Ca^{++} outside the cell account for the negative membrane potential at rest.

Once electrically stimulated, the cellular action potential is initiated and the membrane becomes depolarized (Fig. 10–3). At this time, the electrical stimulation of the cell membrane causes a flow of Na^+ into the cell and a decreased flow of K^+ out. This results in the accumulation of positive ions inside the cell and therefore a less negative membrane potential.

The membrane action potential consists of five phases. The action potential begins with phase 4. This is the resting phase of the cell. Phase 0 begins with the rapid entry of Na^+ into the cell. At phase 1, rapid repolarization represented by a decrease in positive electrical readings inside the cell is initiated with an inward flow of Cl^- and an outward flow of K^+. Phase 2 or the plateau phase represents the inward flow of Ca^{++} and Cl^-. Final repolarization of the membrane or phase 3 occurs with an outward flow of K^+ and a decreased flow of Ca^{++} inward.

Two other features of cardiac cells that relate to membrane potentials and that are important considerations in the formation of arrhythmias are membrane responsiveness and the membrane refractory period. Membrane responsiveness represents that point (the threshold) on the membrane where potential can be initiated. The refractory period is that time frame that occurs once a cardiac cell generates an action potential until the next action potential can be generated.

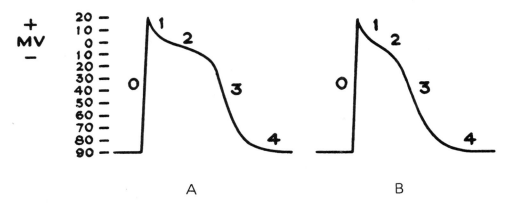

Figure 10–3. Typical action potential for ventricular (**A**) and atrial (**B**) cardiac tissue. (Adapted from Goldman MJ: Principles of Clinical Electrocardiography, 10th ed. Los Altos, Calif, Lange Medical Publications, 1979, with permission.)

Formation of Arrhythmias

Arrhythmias arise from alterations in normal impulse initiation or automaticity or alteration in the normal impulse conduction pattern or both. They usually result in abnormalities in cardiac rate, rhythm, and conduction.

As previously stated, automaticity is defined as the inherent ability of some cardiac cells to depolarize and generate an action potential spontaneously. These cells are primarily located in the SA node. When this tissue fails to initiate an impulse, other secondary or ectopic pacemakers are formed. The formation of

TABLE 10–3. ANTIARRHYTHMIA AGENTS

Generic Name	Trade Name	Mechanism of Action	Route of Administration	Adverse Reactions
Class IA				
quinidine	—	Decreases automaticity and slows conduction in atria and ventricles	PO	Gastrointestinal upsets, thrombocytopenia, rash, hypotension, heart block, tachyarrhythmias, cinchonism
disopyramide	Norpace	Decreases automaticity and increases atrial and ventricular refractoriness	PO	Anticholinergic effects, hypotension, heart failure, tachyarrhythmias, heart block
procainamide	Procan SR, Pronestyl	Same as quinidine	PO, IV	Lupus-like syndrome, central nervous system effects, gastrointestinal upset, rash, hypotension, arrhythmias, blood dyscrasia
Class IB				
lidocaine	—	Increases threshold for electrical stimulation of myocardium	IV, IM	Central nervous system effects, seizures, paresthesias
phenytoin	Dilantin	Depresses spontaneous depolarization in ventricular tissue	PO, IV	Intravenous infusion greater than 50 mg/min associated with cardiac toxicity, toxic effects include slurred speech, ataxia, and nystagmus
tocainide	Tonocard	Same as lidocaine	PO, IV	Central nervous system effects, nausea, anorexia, increased ventricular arrhythmias
Class II				
propanolol	Inderal	Blocks AV node conduction and prolongs refractory period	PO, IV	Heart block, heart failure, hypotension, bronchospasm
acebutolol	Sectral	Same as propanolol	PO	Fatigue, headache, dizziness, diarrhea, gastrointestinal upsets
Class III				
bretylium	Bretylol	Prolongs refractory period	IV, IM	Hypotension, nausea, vomiting, may increase severity of arrhythmia at onset of therapy
Class IV				
verapamil	Isoptin, Calan	Slows conduction through AV node	PO, IV	Heart block, hypotension, bradycardia
Other agents				
digoxin	Lanoxin	Slows conduction through AV node	PO, IV	Arrhythmias, gastrointestinal upsets, fatigue, weakness
atropine sulfate	—	Blocks vagal impulses to the heart	PO, IV IM, SQ	Dry mouth, cycloplegia, mydriasis, urinary retention, constipation, confusion

TABLE 10–4. CHARACTERISTICS OF SOME COMMON CLINICAL ARRHYTHMIAS

Arrhythmia	Atrial Rate (bpm)	Ventricular Rate (bpm)	Rhythm
Sinus tachycardia	100–200	100–200	Regular
Sinus bradycardia	40–60	40–60	Regular
Atrial flutter	240–350	80–150	Regular
Atrial fibrillation	300–600	140–175	Very irregular
Paroxysmal atrial tachycardia	150–250	150–250	Regular
AV nodal tachycardia	180–199	100–180	Regular
Ventricular tachycardia	Variable	100–250	Regular to slightly irregular
Ventricular fibrillation	Variable	300	No pulse present

ectopic pacemakers can lead to a variety of arrhythmias which decrease the heart's ability to deliver oxygenated blood.

The other source of arrhythmia formation consists of alterations in impulse conduction. The normal series of events involved in impulse conduction has already been described. Termination of the impulse occurs after it has traversed the ventricles because the surrounding tissue is in the refractory period. Under certain conditions, however, the impulse does not die but continues to re-excite cardiac tissue. This phenomenon is known as re-entry or circus movement and can occur either in the atrial or ventricular tissue. This re-entry phenomenon can cause either single premature beats or repetitive ectopic beats. Table 10–4 lists common arrhythmias and their descriptions.

Drugs used to treat arrhythmias are given in Table 10–3. They are grouped in classes based on their major electrophysiological properties. Table 10–5 gives the drugs and their indication(s) of use, and Table 10–6 gives the effects of the drugs on the myocardium. Agents that belong to the same class will be discussed together.

TABLE 10–5. INDICATIONS FOR USE OF ANTIARRHYTHMIA AGENTS

Generic Name	Trade Name	Indications
Class IA		
quinidine	—	Atrial, supraventricular arrhythmias, paroxysmal atrial tachycardia, chronic ventricular arrhythmias
disopyramide	Norpace	Premature ventricular contractions, ventricular tachycardia
procainamide	Procan SR Pronestyl	Atrial and supraventricular arrhythmias, paroxysmal atrial fibrillation and tachycardia, ventricular tachycardia, ventricular and atrial premature contractions
Class IB		
lidocaine	—	Ventricular arrhythmias
phenytoin	Dilantin	Parodoxical atrial arrhythmias, ventricular arrhythmias
tocainide	Tonocard	Ventricular arrhythmias
Class II		
propanolol	Inderal	Atrial and supraventricular arrhythmias
acebutolol	Sectral	Same as propanolol
Class III		
bretylium	Bretylol	Ventricular arrhythmias
Class IV		
verapamil	Calan Isoptin	Supraventricular arrhythmias
Other agents		
digoxin	Lanoxin	Atrial fibrillation and flutter, paroxysmal atrial tachycardia
atropine sulfate	—	Bradycardia

TABLE 10–6. CARDIAC ACTIONS OF ANTIARRHYTHMIA AGENTS

Generic Name	Conduction Velocity	Automaticity	Contractility
atropine	Increased	Increased	No change
bretylium	No change	No change or slight increase	No change or slight increase
digoxin	Slowed	Increased	Increased
disopyramide	No change or slightly slowed	Decreased	Decreased
lidocaine	No change	Decreased	No change
phenytoin	No change or slight increase	Decreased	No change
procainamide	Slowed	Decreased	Decreased
propanolol	Slowed	Decreased	Decreased
quinidine	Slowed	Decreased	Decreased
verapamil	Slowed	No change or slight decrease	Decreased

CLASS IA AGENTS

Action and Fate. Quinidine, procainamide, and disopyramide are grouped together as class IA agents. These drugs exert two effects on cardiac tissue: one directly by suppressing myocardial activity (depressing automaticity), the other indirectly by their anticholinergic effect. These agents slightly prolong the duration of the action potential and significantly prolong the refractory period. The anticholinergic effects, which are greater with quinidine and disopyramide, block vagal stimulation of the AV node which in turn increases ventricular rate.

Quinidine is metabolized in the liver and excreted via the kidneys. Ten to 30 percent is excreted unchanged. About 60 percent of procainamide is excreted unchanged; the rest is excreted as an active metabolite. Disopyramide is metabolized in the liver with 40 to 60 percent excreted unchanged.

Uses. The indications for the use of quinidine and procainamide are very similar. They are used to treat premature atrial, AV junctional, and ventricular contractions, paroxysmal atrial tachycardia, ventricular tachycardia, and to maintain normal sinus rhythm after DC cardioversion of atrial flutter or fibrillation. Disopyramide is used to suppress and prevent premature ventricular contractions and tachycardia.

Side and Adverse Effects. Quinidine can cause hypotension and a variety of arrhythmias. It also can cause gastrointestinal upsets and visual disturbances. An idiosyncratic reaction, cinchonism, is caused by quinidine. It consists of ringing in the ears, dizziness, visual disturbances, and vertigo. It can also cause a variety of dermatologic reactions. Procainamide can also produce hypotension, a variety of arrhythmias, and gastrointestinal upset. Agranulocytosis and leukopenia have also been reported. Prolonged use of procainamide can produce a lupus-like syndrome manifested as joint pain, fever, and rash. The side effects associated with disopyramide are primarily gastrointestinal upset, dry mouth, and urinary retention.

Contraindications and Cautions. Quinidine should not be used in any individual who has previously had a hypersensitivity or idiosyncratic reaction (cinchonism) to the drug. It should not be used in complete heart block and should be used cautiously in incomplete heart block. Procainamide should not be used in individuals with second or third degree or complete heart block or blood dyscrasias. Its use should also be avoided in those with or a past history of systemic lupus erythematosus (SLE).

NURSING IMPLICATIONS

Quinidine

- Continuous monitoring of ECG and blood pressure is required when initiating treatment.
- Quinidine can cause the idiosyncratic reaction known as cinchonism (nausea, vomiting, headache, dizziness, fever, tremors, vertigo, visual disturbances, tinnitus). Monitor patient for symptoms. Test dose may be given to determine if patient is prone to reaction.
- Can cause unpredictable rhythm abnormalities in digitalized heart.
- Monitor intake and output. Be alert for electrolyte imbalances due to diarrhea that may occur early in therapy.
- During long-term therapy, periodic blood counts, serum electrolytes, and kidney and liver function tests are advised.
- Increased blood levels of digoxin, necessitating a decrease in digoxin dose.

Procainamide

- Patients with severe heart, hepatic, or renal disease are at higher risk for adverse effects with procainamide.
- When used for atrial arrhythmia, may precipitate ventricular tachycardia.
- Monitor patient for hypotensive effect.
- Apical pulse should be checked prior to each oral dose when drug is first given.
- Lupus erythematosus (LE) test and ANA titer are done at regular intervals when patients are on long-term maintenance dosage.
- Patients should promptly report the onset of SLE-like syndrome symptoms: polyarthralgia, chest pain, cough, fever, and malaise.

Disopyramide

- Use contraindicated in cardiogenic shock or second or third degree heart block with no pacemaker.
- Check apical pulse prior to administration; hold medication and notify health professional if below 60 or above 120.
- Monitor blood pressure.
- Monitor input-output ratio; watch for weight gain.

CLASS IB AGENTS

Action and Fate. Lidocaine and phenytoin are the two class IB agents. Both agents depress automaticity primarily in the Purkinje fibers. The agents can terminate re-entry phenomenon by producing a bidirectional conduction through damage-conducting tissue. At therapeutic doses neither agent produces significant ECG changes.

Both agents are extensively metabolized in the liver and excreted via the kidneys.

Uses. Lidocaine is indicated for control of ventricular arrhythmias occurring during acute myocardial infarction, cardiac surgery, or catheterization and those arrhythmias caused by digitalis toxicity.

Phenytoin, although not approved, is used for treatment of paradoxical atrial tachycardia and ventricular arrhythmias, especially those caused by digitalis toxicity.

Side and Adverse Effects. Lidocaine primarily causes central nervous system side effects such as dizziness, disorientation, confusion, agitation, euphoria, convulsions, and coma.

Phenytoin can cause sedation, nystagmus, ataxia, slurred speech, and gum overgrowth known as gingival hyperplasia.

Contraindications and Cautions. Lidocaine should not be used in individuals with a history of hypersensitivity reactions to related local anesthetics (amide type). It should be used cautiously in those with liver impairment and congestive heart failure.

Phenytoin should not be given to those with complete or incomplete heart block. Cautious use is recommended in individuals with impaired liver function and diabetes mellitus.

NURSING IMPLICATIONS

Phenytoin

- Be alert for ECG signs of excessive cardiac depression, which could lead to heart block.
- Margin between therapeutic and toxic doses is small. Therapeutic blood concentration equals 10 to 20 μg/ml; toxic level equals 30 to 50 μg/ml.
- To give phenytoin parenterally, the preferred means is slow intravenous push not to exceed 50 mg/min; a faster rate can cause heart block. Normal saline is used to flush the line before and after administration; the use of a dextrose containing solution, such as D_5W, will cause precipitation of the drug.

Lidocaine

- Constant ECG monitoring and frequent blood pressure determinations are necessary to avoid potential overdose and toxicity.
- Monitor patient for neurotoxic effects: drowsiness, dizziness, confusion, paresthesias, visual disturbances, excitation, and behavioral changes.
- Reports of convulsions are common.
- Blood levels of 1.5 to 6 μg/ml provide antiarrhythmic activity, levels above 7 μg/ml are potentially toxic.
- Should be discontinued or changed to another antiarrythmic agent if therapeutic effect not achieved within 24 hours.
- Lidocaine is administered as a bolus of 50 to 100 mg IV push, followed as a continuous infusion at a rate of 1 to 2 mg/min.
- Note on label that correct preparation of lidocaine is used; lidocaine for arrhythmias is not the preparation for local anesthesia.

CLASS II AGENTS (BETA BLOCKERS)

Action and Fate. The antiarrhythmic effect of these agents is due mainly to their blockade of beta receptors thus blocking sympathetic stimulation of cardiac tissue.

Uses. The beta blockers are most effective in the treatment of supraventricular arrhythmias that result from an increase of sympathetic influence on the heart as may occur during surgery. The beta blockers may also be used for arrhythmias caused by digitalis toxicity.

Side and Adverse Effects, Contraindications and Cautions, and Nursing Implications. See Hypertensive Agents, in this chapter.

CLASS III AGENTS

Action and Fate. Bretylium is the only agent presently in class III. It is not usually considered an agent of first choice in the treatment of cardiac arrhythmias. Bretylium can suppress ventricular fibrillation, by direct suppression of ventricular tissue and ventricular tachycardia by adrenergic blockade. Adrenergic blockade is not an immediate effect however. Initially bretylium causes the release of norepinephrine from adrenergic postganglionic nerve terminals. This action can cause a transient increase in blood pressure, heart rate, and ventricular irritability. Then both the release and re-uptake of norepinephrine are blocked because the drug causes a depression of adrenergic nerve excitability.

Bretylium is excreted unchanged via the kidneys.

Use. Bretylium is used for short-term treatment of ventricular tachycardia in those who have not responded to other agents.

Side and Adverse Effects. Bretylium can cause hypotension accompanied by dizziness, vertigo, and faintness. It can precipitate angina. Other effects include gastrointestinal upset, shortness of breath, and various dermatologic reactions.

Contraindications and Cautions. Bretylium should not be used for digitalis-induced arrhythmias or severe hypotension. It should be used cautiously in kidney impairment and in those on digitalis.

NURSING IMPLICATIONS

* Blood pressure and heart function are constantly monitored during the use of bretylium.
* Monitor patient closely for initial transient rise in blood pressure, increased heart rate, and arrhythmias, or worsening of existing arrhythmias.
* Initial rise in blood pressure is usually followed by a fall in blood pressure in about an hour after time of administration.
* Instruct patient to remain supine until tolerant to hypotensive effect of bretylium.
* The administration of bretylium intravenously is associated with a high evidence of nausea and vomiting.

CLASS IV AGENTS (CALCIUM CHANNEL BLOCKERS)

See Calcium Channel Blockers, in this chapter.

MISCELLANEOUS AGENTS

Two other agents used to manage arrhythmias are digoxin and atropine. Digoxin is indicated in the treatment of supraventricular tachycardias such as atrial fibrillation, atrial flutter, and paroxysmal atrial tachycardia. For more information, see previous section on Cardiac Glycosides in this chapter.

Atropine, as an anticholinergic agent, blocks all vagal tone to the heart. Its use is indicated in cardiac arrest and to reverse bradycardia induced by beta-blocking agents and cholinergic drugs.

When administering atropine, the patient's vital signs should be monitored. Note quality and rate of pulse, respiration, and changes in blood pressure and temperature. Report any deviations from the normal. Following intravenous administration of atropine, there may be a paradoxical bradycardia, which usually lasts 1 to 2 minutes. Atropine can cause urinary retention. For this reason a urinary output baseline should be established and monitored during therapy. Atropine also causes constipation; laxatives or a dietary change can relieve the problem. The dry mouth that occurs can be relieved by mouth rinses with water or artificial saliva. The elderly are prone to "atropine fever" caused by perspiration and heat loss suppression. This puts these particular patients at risk for heat stroke. Advice the patient to avoid excessive heat. Intraocular pressure should be measured before and during treatment; if there is an increase, the drug should be discontinued.

Antianginal Agents

Angina pectoris is the most prevalent form of heart disease. It is caused primarily by a narrowing of the coronary arteries. This narrowing of the coronary arteries results in a decreased blood flow to the myocardium. Therefore, when the workload increases, there is an increased demand for oxygen by the myocardium. The demand exceeds the supply and the individual experiences the symptoms associated with angina. In addition to pain, which may radiate to the lower jaw and upper neck and to the inner surface of the arm and down the wrist, hand, and fingers, the individual will also feel anxiety, shortness of breath, diaphoresis, nausea, and vomiting. Angina pectoris is divided into three types. Classic or stable angina is associated with coronary atherosclerosis. An attack is precipitated by exertion, stress, or by eating. The attack is terminated by rest or nitrates. Unstable angina pectoris is a progressive form of the disease, with attacks becoming more severe and more frequent. The attack may even appear during rest. The last type of angina is vasospastic or Prinzmetal's angina. This form of angina is associated with spasms of the coronary arteries and is treated with a calcium channel blocker.

Treatment of angina is divided into relief of acute attacks or the prophylactic management of angina. Termination of acute attacks is managed by the sublingual administration of a nitrate; long-term prophylaxis is usually managed by giving a nitrate (orally or topically), a beta blocker for classic angina, or a calcium channel blocker for variant or Prinzmetal's angina.

NITRATES

Action and Fate. The basic therapeutic action of the nitrates is due to the ability of these agents to relax vascular smooth muscles. This dilates the coronary arteries, which in turn reduces the cardiac workload and myocardial demand for oxygen. This action terminates the pain associated with an anginal attack.

All the nitrates are rapidly metabolized in the liver and excreted in the urine as inactive metabolites.

Uses. The nitrates come in a variety of dosage forms: sublingual tablets, tablets, sustained release tablets or capsules, topical ointment, transdermal patches, IV form, and the most recent addition, the sublingual metered aerosol.

The sublingual tablets and metered aerosol are used to treat acute anginal attacks. They can also be taken prior to an exertional activity as a prophylactic measure. The sustained release tablets or capsules are used as prophylactic measures. Their effectiveness, however, may be limited due to the extensive hepatic metabolism these agents undergo (first-pass effect). The topical ointment is used also as a prophylactic measure, as is the transdermal patch. The IV form is used to relieve anginal pain in individuals refractory to normal doses of nitrates. It is also used as an antihypertensive during specific cardiovascular procedures.

Side and Adverse Effects. The more frequently encountered side effects are related to the vasodilatation produced by these agents. These include headache, dizziness, flushing, postural hypotension, tachycardia, and syncope. Hypersensitivity reactions such as skin rash and dermatitis may also be observed.

Contraindications and Cautions. The use of nitrates is contraindicated in those individuals with known hypersensitivity to these agents. They are also contraindicated in early myocardial infarct. They should be used cautiously in those with hepatic dysfunction.

NURSING IMPLICATIONS

Nitroglycerin Oral

- Sublingual tablets should be placed under the tongue and NOT chewed for best absorption. Patient should be advised to sit or lie down when taking nitroglycerin. If pain is relieved completely, any remaining tablet can be expelled from the mouth. If pain is not relieved, repeat after 5 minutes for two times more. If pain persists, this may indicate an acute myocardial infarct. Patient should contact physician immediately or go to an emergency room.
- Tablet should pop or give a stinging sensation under the tongue if potent. Headache, dizziness, and syncope are frequent side effects; may last approximately 20 minutes.
- Tablets should be kept in original amber glass container; exposure to air, light, humidity, and heat will hasten their deterioration. Therefore, unused tablets should be discarded 6 months after bottle is opened and a new supply obtained.
- Tablets can be taken prophylactically prior to any exertive activity, e.g., sex, exercise.
- Sustained oral release formulations are taken on an empty stomach with a full glass of water and swallowed whole. These agents are used prophylactically to prevent anginal attacks. Their use is not intended for relief of acute attacks.

Nitroglycerin Topical

- Ointment is measured on a special applicator pad by inches and applied in a thin uniform layer. Do not use fingers to spread because the administrator will also absorb the drug.
- Once applied, the ointment may be covered with plastic wrap to protect clothing.
- Areas commonly used for application are chest, abdomen, and forearm.
- Observe application sights for inflammation and sensitization due to allergic reaction to ointment base.
- Transdermal system releases a controlled amount of nitroglycerin over a 24-hour period (see Table 10–8 for various preparations).
- Application of the patch is usually on the chest. Excessive hair on application area should be clipped, not shaven. Shaving area will alter the amount of nitroglycerin absorbed.
- Contact with water does not effect the patch.
- Instruct patient to remove old patch before applying new patch.
- Observe application site for inflammation and sensitization due to allergic reaction to adhesive.

TABLE 10–7. VARIOUS NITROGLYCERIN PRODUCTS AND THEIR ROUTES OF ADMINISTRATION

Generic Name	Trade Name	Route of Administration
amyl nitrate	—	Inhalation
erythrityl tetranitrate	Cardilate	Sublingual, oral
isosorbide dinitrate	Isordil Sorbitrate	Sublingual, oral
nitroglycerin	Various	Sublingual, oral, topical, intravenous
pentaerythritol tetranitrate	P.E.T.N. Peritrate	Oral

TABLE 10–8. COMPARISON OF THE VARIOUS NITROGLYCERIN PATCHES[a]

Trade Name	Manufacturer	Patch Size (cm²)	Average Amount of Nitroglycerin Delivered in 24 hr
Transderm-Nitro 2.5	Ciba	5	2.5 mg
Nitro-Dur 5	Key	5	2.5 mg
Nitrodisc 5	Searle	8	5.0 mg
Transderm-Nitro 5	Ciba	10	5.9 mg
Nitro-Dur 10	Key	10	5.0 mg
Nitro-Dur 15	Key	15	7.5 mg
Nitrodisc 10	Searle	16	10.0 mg
Transderm-Nitro 10	Ciba	20	10.0 mg
Nitro-Dur 20	Key	20	10.0 mg
Transderm-Nitro 15	Ciba	30	15.0 mg

[a] Shows the differences in the amount of drug delivered in a 24-hour period. Note that not all products are equivalent.

Nitroglycerin Intravenous

- Nitroglycerin for intravenous use must be diluted in either D_5W or NS prior to infusion.
- Use only glass containers for dilution and nonpolyvinylchloride IV tubing.
- IV infusion of nitroglycerin requires continuous monitoring of blood pressure and heart rate.

NON-NITRATES

Beta Receptor Blockers

Beta receptor blockers may be used as prophylactic agents in the management of angina. These agents reduce blood pressure, cardiac workload, and oxygen consumption by the myocardium. A detailed discussion of the beta receptor blockers is given in this chapter under Antihypertensive Agents.

Calcium Channel Blocking Agents

Calcium channel blocking agents are effective in preventing recurring anginal pain of the variant or Prinzmetal type. These agents inhibit the influx of calcium ions into the myocardium decreasing cardiac muscle contractibility. They also dilate coronary arteries. These effects reduce cardiac workload thus decreasing myocardial demand for oxygen. A detailed discussion of calcium channel blockers is given in the section on Calcium Channel Blockers in this chapter.

Antihypertensive Agents

Hypertension or high blood pressure is defined as a blood pressure reading in excess of 140/90 mm Hg recorded at three separate times. It is also known as the silent killer since there are no specific symptoms associated with this disease that could alert the affected individual. In addition, if left untreated or inadequately treated, the long-term consequences involve damage to one or more of the target organ systems, i.e., heart, brain, kidneys, and eyes. Increased blood pressure

TABLE 10–9. ANTIHYPERTENSIVE AGENTS

Generic Name	Trade Name	Maximum Daily Dose[a]
Thiazide diuretics[b]		
Sympatholytic agents		
Centrally acting		
clonidine	Catapres	2.4 mg
methyldopa	Aldomet	2 Gm
Centrally and peripherally acting		
reserpine	Serpasil	0.25 mg
Neurotransmission blocker		
guanethidine	Ismelin	200 mg
Beta receptor blockers		
metoprolol	Lopressor	200 mg
propranolol	Inderal	480 mg
Alpha receptor blocker		
prazosin	Minipress	20 mg
Angiotensin-converting enzyme inhibitor		
captopril	Capoten	300 mg
Direct-acting vasodilator		
hydralazine	Apresoline	50 mg
minoxidil	Loniten	100 mg

[a] Maximum dose usually divided and given twice or three times a day.
[b] See the following section, Diuretics, for information on thiazide diuretics.

leads to an increased workload on the heart that contributes to angina, heart failure, and myocardial infarct. Individuals with hypertension tend to have a higher incidence of strokes than normotensive individuals. Uncontrolled hypertension can cause renal failure and retinal damage in the eye. Early detection and treatment will decrease the risk of these consequences of hypertension and increase life expectancy.

In some cases there are specific underlying causes of hypertension such as pheochromocytoma or hyperthyroidism. Once the underlying condition is corrected, blood pressure returns to normal. This secondary type of hypertension accounts for only a small percent of the cases. Usually a specific underlying cause or a precipitating factor cannot be identified. This is known as essential or idiopathic hypertension. It is thought that this type of hypertension is caused by a combination of several factors, both environmental and genetic in origin (Table 10–10). If an individual is diagnosed as a borderline hypertensive (diastolic not above 90 mm Hg), nonpharmacological interventions are usually employed (Table 10–11). If this approach is not sufficient or if the diastolic pressure measures above 90 mm Hg, the stepwise therapeutic approach is used as recommended by the Joint National Committee on Detection, Evaluation and Treatment of High Blood Pressure. This is one of the few treatment regimens in which multidrug therapy is considered to be a rational approach in disease management.

TABLE 10–10. FACTORS THAT MAY CONTRIBUTE TO THE DEVELOPMENT OF HYPERTENSION

Genetic make-up of the individual

Race

Stress

Sedentary life style

Excessive sodium intake

Excessive caffeine intake

Excessive weight

Tobacco use

Alcohol use

Use of stimulant drugs

TABLE 10–11. SUMMARY OF SOME NONPHARMACOLOGICAL APPROACHES IN THE TREATMENT OF IDIOPATHIC HYPERTENSION

Sodium-restricted diet

Caffeine-restricted intake

Weight reduction if overweight

Tobacco use reduction or restriction

Relaxation techniques

Supervised exercise

The various classes of drugs used in this stepwise regimen are diuretics, sympatholytic agents, vasodilators, and angiotensin-converting enzyme inhibitors. Therapy is usually initiated with a thiazide diuretic. In some cases, therapy may be started with a beta blocker if the blood pressure is caused by high blood levels of renin. If a diuretic alone does not adequately lower blood pressure, then one of the drugs from Step 2 is added to the regimen. Again, if blood pressure is not normalized, the Step 3 agent can be added to the regimen. Step 4 agents are used if the blood pressure remains elevated. If a Step 4 agent is needed, then the Step 3 agent may or may not be discontinued. As a rule, drugs in the same step are usually not used simultaneously; however, there may be exceptions in refractory individuals (Fig. 10–4).

Since this therapeutic class of agents consists of various types of drugs, each class will be individually discussed and summarized in the tables. Information concerning diuretics will not be repeated and the reader is referred to Diuretics in this chapter.

SYMPATHOLYTIC AGENTS

Beta Blockers

Action and Fate. Beta blockers compete with both epinephrine and norepinephrine for beta receptor sites. Most beta-blocking agents interact with both

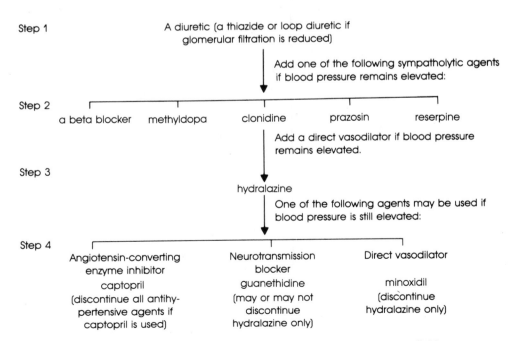

Figure 10–4. Stepwise therapeutic approach to the management of essential hypertension used when the nonpharmacological interventions do not normalize the blood pressure. Deviations may occur from this scheme depending on the individual case.

TABLE 10–12. BETA BLOCKERS AND THEIR CARDIOSELECTIVE ACTION

Generic Name	Trade Name	Cardioselective Action
acebutolol	Sectral	Yes
atenolol	Tenormin	Yes
labetalol	Normodyne	No
metoprolol	Lopressor	Yes
nadolol	Corgard	No
pindolol	Visken	No
propranolol	Inderal	No
timolol	Blocadren	No
	Timoptic[a]	

[a] Timoptic ophthalmic drops used to control glaucoma.

the cardiac (beta 1) receptors and the bronchial (beta 2) receptors. Some agents may be somewhat more selective in blocking beta 1 receptors (Table 10–12). All beta blockers lower blood pressure by decreasing cardiac output and suppressing renin activity.

Beta blockers are excreted in different ways. Metoprolol is metabolized in the liver and excreted via the kidney. Atenolol and nadolol are excreted unchanged via the kidneys. Pindolol, propranolol, and timolol are excreted both unchanged and as metabolites.

Uses. All the beta blockers are used primarily as Step 2 agents along with a diuretic in the management of hypertension. In addition, propranolol is also used for the treatment of cardiac arrhythmias, thyrotoxicosis, and pheochromocytoma. Other uses of propranolol include prevention of migraine headaches and panic attacks.

Side and Adverse Effects. Side effects associated with the use of beta blockers include bronchospasm especially in those individuals with a history of bronchoconstrictive diseases. These agents can also cause hypoglycemia in addition to masking its adrenergic symptoms. Other side effects include bradycardia (pulse below 60/min), central nervous system effects such as dizziness, fatigue, mental confusion, depression, and insomnia.

Contraindications and Cautions. Use of beta blockers should be avoided in individuals with greater than first degree heart block, CHF, and bronchoconstrictive diseases such as asthma, chronic obstructive pulmonary disease (COPD), and allergic rhinitis. Cautious use is indicated in diabetes, peripheral vascular diseases, and renal and hepatic impairment.

NURSING IMPLICATIONS

- Use with extreme care in patients with asthma; may cause serious and even fatal bronchial spasms.
- If signs and symptoms of bronchoconstriction are noted, hold medication and call physician.
- Use with extreme caution in CHF as decreased heart rate may result in acute cardiac decompensation and worsen CHF.
- Observe the ECG, central venous pressure (CVP), heart rate, and blood pressure when administering IV. Stop if heart rate increases or decreases.
- Note and report patients who develop bradycardia. May be reversed with atropine.
- Oral dose may cause gastrointestinal upset; may be best to give with meals.
- Check IV placement prior to administering. GIVE IV SLOWLY.

- May cause water and sodium retention.
- HOLD DRUG if heart rate is less than 60 apical or systolic blood pressure is less than 90; call physician.
- Monitor diabetic patients carefully; drug may cause and mask signs of hypoglycemia.
- Advise patient NOT to discontinue drug abruptly; it must be withdrawn over a 48-hour period. Abrupt discontinuation may cause a fatal heart attack or precipitate arrhythmias.

Alpha Receptor Blocker

Action and Fate. The only alpha receptor blocking agent currently available for the long-term management of hypertension is prazosin. It is thought to cause a peripheral vasodilatation by blocking alpha receptors located mainly on the arterioles. As a result, this agent reduces orthostatic and supine blood pressure with the greater lowering effect being on the diastolic pressure.

The drug is probably metabolized in the liver and excreted in the bile and feces; a small amount is excreted in the urine.

Use. Prazosin is used in conjunction with a diuretic and is considered a Step 2 agent in the management of hypertension.

Side and Adverse Effects. The initial dose of prazosin, if greater than 1 mg, is associated with a transient feeling of lightheadedness, dizziness, weakness, and syncope. These symptoms are known as the "first dose phenomenon." For this reason the dose should be increased gradually to the effective dose. Some gastrointestinal effects may also be experienced such as vomiting, diarrhea, and abdominal discomfort.

Contraindications and Cautions. Prazosin should be used cautiously in individuals with kidney or liver dysfunction. Safe use in women during pregnancy or lactating, or during childbearing age not established.

NURSING IMPLICATIONS

- Food may delay absorption, but does not effect degree of absorption.
- "First dose phenomenon," a transient, dose-related syndrome manifested by dizziness, weakness, lightheadedness, and syncope may occur 30 minutes to 2 hours after initial dose. Assist patient with any changes of position.

Centrally Acting Agents

Action and Fate. The centrally acting agents are clonidine and methyldopa. Clonidine acts to lower blood pressure by interacting with the preganglionic alpha$_2$ (α_2) receptors to produce an inhibition of sympathetic outflow from the vasomotor centers. This reduces the peripheral sympathetic nervous system activity, lowers the systolic and diastolic blood pressure, and decreases heart rate. A portion of clonidine is metabolized in the liver and both nonmetabolized drug and metabolites are excreted via the kidneys.

The exact mechanism of action of methyldopa is not known. It is structurally related to the catecholamines and related molecules and may act as a false neurotransmitter. The drug appears to affect both the central and peripheral nervous systems by displacing norepinephrine from storage granules in neurons. Methyldopa is metabolized in the gastrointestinal tract and liver and is excreted via the kidneys. Methyldopa crosses the placenta and is found in breast milk.

Uses. Both agents are Step 2 agents and are used with a diuretic in the treatment of mild hypertension and in conjunction with Step 3 or 4 agents for severe hypertension. Methyldopa is preferred in those individuals with renal failure.

Side and Adverse Effects. Clonidine causes some anticholinergic side effects such as drowsiness, dry mouth, and constipation. Other side effects include orthostatic hypotension and a rebound hypertension if the drug is abruptly discontinued. Methyldopa causes daytime sedation, decreased mental alertness, depression, dry mouth, sexual dysfunction, and hemolytic anemia.

Contraindications and Cautions. The safe use of clonidine during pregnancy and during the childbearing years in women has not been established. Cautious use is recommended in severe coronary insufficiency, recent myocardial infarction, cerebrovascular disease, chronic renal failure, and a history of depression.

NURSING IMPLICATIONS

Methyldopa

- Side effects include depression, tiredness, impotency, dry mouth, dark urine, nightmares, and drowsiness.
- Take at night secondary to drowsiness effect.
- Take blood pressure prior to administration; hold if systolic less than 110 and call physician.
- May cause blood dyscrasias and positive Coomb's test.

Clonidine

- Side effects include drowsiness, dry mouth, constipation. Instruct patient to notify physician if side effects occur.
- If drug is stopped suddenly, restlessness, insomnia, increased salivation, tachycardia, abdominal pain, nausea, and severe hypertensive crisis can occur.

Peripherally Acting Agents

Action and Fate. The two agents that are peripheral vasodilators are reserpine and guanethidine. Reserpine is a natural substance extracted from the Indian snake root plant *Rauwolfia serpentina*. Reserpine first acts to deplete norepinephrine and serotonin from their respective storage granules in neurons found in the brain and peripheral nervous system. Then the drug enters the storage granules preventing the storage of the two neurotransmitters. Reserpine is extensively metabolized in the liver and excreted via the kidneys and feces. It crosses the placenta and appears in breast milk.

Guanethidine depletes norepinephrine at postganglionic neurons by preventing the re-uptake of the neurotransmitters. This interference with neurotransmission causes an arteriolar vasodilatation. Guanethidine is principally excreted via the kidneys as unmetabolized drug.

Uses. Reserpine is indicated in mild hypertension as a Step 2 agent. It is usually combined with a diuretic. Guanethidine is a Step 4 agent and is usually used in conjunction with a diuretic and a Step 2 agent. Hydralazine (Step 4 agent) may be retained or discontinued if guanethidine is added to the regimen.

Side and Adverse Effects. Guanethidine causes orthostatic hypotension, diarrhea, ejaculation problems, and tachycardia. Reserpine is responsible for causing a variety of side effects. Among them are nasal congestion, sedation, lethargy, severe depression, sodium and water retention, nightmares, peptic ulcers, and decreased libido.

Contraindications and Cautions. Guanethidine is contraindicated in CHF and used cautiously in those with diabetes mellitus and impaired renal function. Reserpine should be used in individuals with a history of mental depression or peptic ulcer disease. Safe use during pregnancy and in women of childbearing ages has not been established for either agent.

NURSING IMPLICATIONS

Reserpine

- Administer with milk or food to avoid gastric upset.
- Side effects include drowsiness, sedation, and dizziness; teach patient the importance of reporting these to physician.
- Serious mental depression that may lead to suicide in high doses. Instruct patient and family to report symptoms of depression, anorexia, and mood swings immediately to physician.

Guanethidine

- Dosage adjustments for guanethidine are made for each individual patient based on orthostatic and supine blood pressure readings.
- There is a high incidence of orthostatic and exertional hypotension with dizziness, lightheadedness, and fainting. For this reason, caution patients to change positions slowly and not to get out of bed without assistance.
- Advise patients to report any change of frequency and consistency of stools. Constipation or explosive diarrhea can occur.
- The 10-mg tablets contain tartrazine, which causes allergic reactions including bronchial asthma in susceptible individuals.
- Due to the sexual dysfunction that guanethidine causes in males, these patients may need supportive assistance.

DIRECT VASODILATORS

Action and Fate. The two antihypertensive agents classed as direct vasodilators are hydralazine and minoxidil. Hydralazine acts by direct relaxation of vascular smooth muscle with greater effect on the arterioles. This results in a greater effect on the diastolic pressure than on the systolic pressure. The drug is metabolized in the liver and intestinal wall then excreted via the kidneys.

Minoxidil is also a direct vasodilator but with a more potent hypotensive effect than hydralazine. It also has a greater relaxation effect on the arterioles. Minoxidil is metabolized in the liver and excreted via the kidneys and feces.

Uses. Hydralazine is considered a Step 3 agent in the management of hypertension. Minoxidil is used as a Step 4 agent. Both agents are used in conjunction with a diuretic and are also usually used with a beta blocker to control the reflex tachycardia produced by both.

Side and Adverse Effects. The use of both agents is commonly associated with cardiovascular effects such as palpitations, angina, and tachycardia. Also, some orthostatic hypotension may occur, especially with hydralazine. Other side effects of hydralazine include gastrointestinal effects (anorexia, nausea, vomiting) and a systemic lupus erythematosus syndrome. Minoxidil can cause hypertrichosis (excessive hair growth). Both agents cause sodium and water retention.

Contraindications and Cautions. The use of hydralazine is contraindicated in individuals with lupus erythematosus and angina. Cautious use is indicated in those with liver dysfunction. Minoxidil is contraindicated in those with pheochromocytoma. Cautious use in those with renal or liver dysfunction, angina, and in those who have had a recent myocardial infarct. Safe use during pregnancy has not been established for either agent.

NURSING IMPLICATIONS

Minoxidil

- Intake and output and daily weights should be monitored to ascertain if patient is retaining fluids.
- Blood pressure and apical pulse should be taken prior to administration.
- Patients should take apical pulse at home and report an increase of 20 bpm or more in addition to reporting weight gain and difficulty in breathing.
- Patients should be informed of the possibility of hypertrichosis: elongation and thickening of hair, especially on the face, arms, and back.

Hydralazine

- Instruct patient to monitor self for edema.
- Long-term use of hydralazine can induce a lupus-like syndrome. LE testing and ANA titer should be done regularly.
- Teach patient to recognize LE symptoms: Polyarthralgia, chest pain, cough, fever, and malaise, and to report them promptly.
- Caution patient to make postural changes slowly because of the possibility of postural hypotension.

ANGIOTENSIN-CONVERTING ENZYME (ACE) INHIBITOR: CAPTOPRIL

Action and Fate. Captopril represents a new class of agents used to control hypertension. The mechanism by which it lowers blood pressure is by inhibiting the action of the enzyme responsible for converting angiotensin I to angiotensin II, a potent vasoconstrictor (Fig. 10–5). This action lowers peripheral vascular resistance and decreases the amount of circulatory aldosterone.

A high percentage (40 to 50 percent) of the drug is excreted unchanged; the remainder is excreted as metabolites. The drug does distribute into the breast milk.

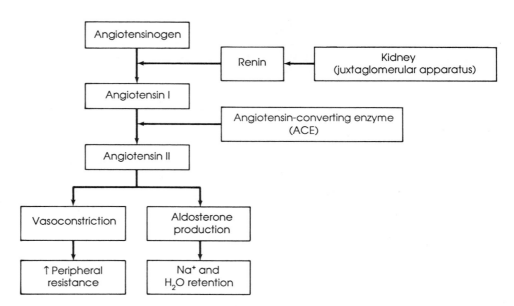

Figure 10–5. Steps in the renin/angiotensin/aldosterone system. ACE inhibitor (Captopril) inhibits the conversion of angiotensin I to angiotensin II.

Uses. Captopril is used as a Step 4 agent in severe hypertension. It may also be used with a cardiac glycoside and diuretics in the treatment of severe edema or congestive heart failure.

Side and Adverse Effects. Captopril causes several important side effects. These include a maculopapular skin rash which usually appears on the upper extremities and trunk. Other side effects include severe anorexia, gastrointestinal distress, a transient agustia (loss of taste sensation), and proteinuria.

Contraindications and Cautions. Captopril should be used with caution in those with renal dysfunction and autoimmune diseases. Safe use in nursing mothers and children not established.

NURSING IMPLICATIONS

- Bedrest is recommended for the first 3 hours of initial administration; blood pressure should be monitored as this medication can cause a hypotensive effect.
- Mild skin eruptions may appear in the first 4 weeks of therapy and may be accompanied by fever. Darkening and crumbling of the nailbeds may also occur. Report to physician if this occurs.
- Taste impairment (dysgeusia) occurs in 5 to 10 percent of patients and usually reverses in 2 to 3 months.

GENERAL NURSING IMPLICATIONS FOR HYPERTENSIVE PATIENTS

- Teach patient to lose weight, decrease fats and salt intake.
- Patients may not feel well on these medications and may refuse to take them. Teach them to call the physician if side effects occur and not to stop taking medications without medical supervision as this may result in hypertensive crisis, CVA, or myocardial infarct.
- Postural hypotension may occur especially with vasodilators. Teach patient to change positions slowly especially from a sitting to standing position.
- Table 10–13 gives the onset of action of several antihypertensive agents given by the oral and intravenous route. These data are important in assessing the response to the medication of an individual whose blood pressure is elevated.
- Teach patient to take own blood pressure daily. Blood pressure should be taken in the same arm (sitting, lying, and standing).
- Supervise ambulation of the elderly taking vasodilators.
- Teach patient to be aware of substances that potentiate the effects of these drugs (narcotics, barbiturates, central nervous system depressants, diuretics, and alcohol).

TABLE 10–13. ONSET OF ACTION OF ANTIHYPERTENSIVE AGENTS

Agent	Onset of Action (Oral)	Onset of Action (Intravenous)
captopril	15 min	—
clonidine	30–60 min	—
guanethidine	Patient must be titrated for maximum effectiveness	—
hydralazine	20–30 min	10–30 min
methyldopa	Slow	4–6 hr
prazosin	2 hr	—
propanolol	30 min	2 min
reserpine	3–6 days	—

- Clear all over-the-counter drugs with a health professional.
- Obtain daily weights and report a gain of 2 lb or more to physician. Be alert to signs and symptoms of fluid overload (central and peripheral edema, profuse rates, S_3 and S_4 heart sounds, and moist cough).
- Monitor input–output ratio; be alert to fluid and electrolyte imbalances.
- Teach patient never to play "catch-up" with hypertensive drugs.
- Always check baseline information on each individual patient. What may be normal blood pressure for one person may be extremely hypertensive for another.
- Encourage the individual to stop smoking, as nicotine is a vasoconstrictor.

Diuretics

There are a number of conditions in which the reduction of excessive body fluid is an essential part of the therapeutic scheme, or in which reduction of excessive fluid gives the individual an improved sense of well-being. The condition could be a chronic one such as CHF or an acute condition such as the elimination of fluid that causes premenstrual edema in some women.

The mechanism by which water and small molecules diffuse through the renal tubule cells and enter the glomerular filtrate is passive diffusion. As the filtrate moves through the nephron, a large percentage of the water and small molecules is reabsorbed (Table 10–14).

In the proximal tubule cells, carbon dioxide (CO_2) is converted to bicarbonate by the enzyme carbonic anhydrase. Bicarbonate is then reabsorbed as sodium bicarbonate ($NaHCO_3$). Also at this site, water and chloride ions (Cl^-) are reabsorbed. The ascending loop of Henle is another site where sodium is reabsorbed. At the distal tubule, sodium ions are actively reabsorbed in exchange for potassium ions (K^+) and they are also reabsorbed in the collection duct in exchange for hydrogen ions (H^+). At each of these sites where sodium ions are reabsorbed, water is also reabsorbed.

By knowing that water passively follows sodium ions in the reabsorption process, it is reasonable to expect that if sodium reabsorption is blocked so will the reabsorption of water. Another means of limiting the amount of water reabsorbed would be to block the action of aldosterone, a hormone, which causes sodium reabsorption. This would block sodium reabsorption in the distal tubule and collecting duct. A third way to limit sodium reabsorption and increase the volume of urine is to increase the osmolarity of the urine. This would lead to more water being retained in the kidney tubule independent of sodium reab-

TABLE 10–14. REABSORPTION OF SUBSTANCES FOUND IN GLOMERULAR FILTRATE

Substances Found in Glomerular Filtrate	% Reabsorbed
Sodium ions (Na^+)	99.4
Chloride ions (Cl^-)	99.2
Bicarbonate ions (HCO_3^-)	100.0
Urea	53.0
Glucose	100.0
Hydrogen ions (H^-)	99.4
Potassium ions (K^+)	100.0
H_2O	99.4

TABLE 10–15. THIAZIDE AND RELATED DIURETICS

Generic Name	Trade Name	Route of Administration	Usual Daily Dose (mg)
bendroflumethiazide	Naturetin	PO	5–20
benzthiazide	Exna	PO	50–200
chlorothiazide	Diuril	PO, IV	500–100
cyclothiazide	Anhydron	PO	1–2
hydrochlorothiazide	Esidrex HydroDiuril Oretic	PO	50–100
hydroflumethiazide	Saluron	PO	20–200
methyclothiazide	Enduron	PO	2.5–10
polythiazide	Renese	PO	1–4
trichlormethiazide	Naqua	PO	2–4
thiazide-like diuretics[a]			
chlorthalidone	Hygroton	PO	25–199
metolazone[b]	Diulo Zaroxolyn	PO	2.5–20
quinethazone	Hydromox	PO	50–100

[a] These are not thiazide diuretics, but they have a similar pharmacology and have been traditionally placed in this class.
[b] This agent has a better diuretic effect than the other agents listed for individuals with renal failure.

sorption. These means of increasing urine output are basic ways in which diuretics act.

There are several classes of diuretics that will be discussed in this unit. They are the osmotic diuretics, a carbonic anhydrase inhibitor, the thiazide diuretics, the loop diuretics, and an aldosterone antagonist. The relative effectiveness of each class of diuretic depends on the amount of sodium prevented from being reabsorbed and varies from mild to potent (Tables 10–15 through 10–17).

OSMOTIC DIURETICS

Action and Fate. Two osmotic diuretics are mannitol and urea. Both agents induce diuresis by raising osmotic pressure of the glomerular filtrate, thus inhibiting renal tubular reabsorption of water. Both agents will also reduce elevated intraocular pressure and elevated cerebrospinal pressure by increasing the plasma osmolarity. This forces water to migrate from regions of low density to those of high density.

Both agents are excreted by the kidneys unchanged by glomerular filtration. For urea, about 50 percent of the drug may be reabsorbed. It also crosses the placenta and is found in breast milk.

TABLE 10–16. LOOP DIURETICS: ROUTES OF ADMINISTRATION AND TIME OF ONSET

Generic Name	Trade Name	Route of Administration	Onset of Action
bumetanide	Bumex	PO	30–60 min
		IM	40 min
		IV	within minutes
ethacrynic acid	Edecrin	PO	30 min
		IV	5 min
furosemide	Lasix	PO	30–60 min
		IM	5 min
		IV	5 min

TABLE 10-17. OTHER DIURETIC AGENTS

Generic Name	Trade Name	Route of Administration
Potassium-sparing agents		
spironolactone	Aldactone	PO
triamterene[a]	Dyrenium	PO
mannitol	Osmitrol	IV
urea		IV (also topical, intra-abdominal, and intra-amniotic)
Carbonic acid anhydrase inhibitor		
acetazolamide	Diamox	PO, IM, IV

[a] Usually used in combination with hydrochlorothiazide.

Uses. Both agents are used to correct certain states of edema not caused by an excessive amount of sodium. Mannitol is used to prevent and treat oliguria in acute renal failure, to reduce edema associated with cardiovascular surgery, to reduce intraocular pressure, to alleviate pulmonary edema, and to enhance excretion of toxic substances. Urea is used to reduce intraocular pressure and to reduce cerebral edema. Administered transabdominally, urea is used as an aborifacient.

Side and Adverse Effects. The use of mannitol is associated with dry mouth, thirst, excessive diuresis, headache, circulatory overload with pulmonary edema, and thrombophlebitis at the infusion site.

Urea is associated with drowsiness, headache, acute psychosis, and fluid and electrolyte imbalances.

Contraindications and Cautions. These agents should not be used in individuals with anuria, severe pulmonary edema, CHF, or severe dehydration.

NURSING IMPLICATIONS

• Serum and urine electrolytes (Na$^+$, K$^+$, Cl$^-$), central venous pressure, and renal function should be closely monitored during therapy.
• Intake and output must be accurately measured and recorded to achieve proper fluid balance. Increasing oliguria is an indication to terminate therapy; report immediately. If urinary output is not adequate, mannitol may accumulate and cause circulatory overload, with resulting edema, water intoxication, and CHF.
• Daily weights are a good indicator of fluid loss or fluid retention.
• Monitor vital signs and be alert for indications of fluid and electrolyte imbalance (e.g., thirst, muscle cramps or weakness, paresthesias) and signs of CHF (jugular venous distention [JVD], dyspnea, rales, tachycardia, and blood pressure changes).

CARBONIC ANHYDRASE INHIBITOR

Action and Fate. The agent in this class of diuretics is acetazolamide. It is a sulfonamide derivative without bacteriostatic action. Its diuretic action is due to its ability to inhibit the action of the enzyme carbonic anhydrase in the proximal renal tubule cells (Fig. 10-6). This action prevents the formation of carbonic acid (H_2CO_3) which is the source of hydrogen (H$^+$) and bicarbonate (HCO$_3^-$) ions. Absence of H$^+$ inhibits renal tubular reabsorption of sodium (Fig. 10-7).

Carbonic anhydrase is also located in two other tissues in the eye and in the central nervous system. Inhibition of the enzyme in the eye prevents the formation of aqueous humor, and in the central nervous system this agent prevents or

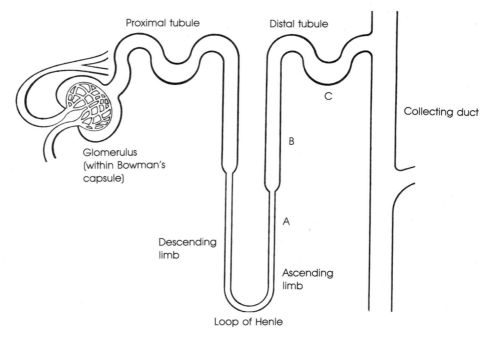

Figure 10–6. The nephron and its functional subdivisions showing the site of action of the major classes of diuretics. At sites A and B (the ascending loop of Henle): loop diuretics. At site B (distal portion of the ascending loop of Henle): thiazide and thiazide-like diuretics. At site C (distal tubule): potassium-sparing diuretics. *(Adapted from Edema and Hypertension: Physiology and Treatment, module I. University of Wisconsin Extension School of Pharmacy, Center for Health Sciences, University of Wisconsin, Madison, Wisconsin, with permission.)*

slows abnormal neuronal discharges by causing neural tissue membrane stabilization.

Acetazolamide penetrates the central nervous system, passes through the placenta, and is excreted unchanged.

Uses. Acetazolamide is used to decrease edema associated with various diseases. It is also used to treat several forms of epilepsy (absence, tonic/clonic, and focal seizures). Acetazolamide is also used to reduce intraocular pressure in open- and closed-angle glaucoma. It may also be used to correct metabolic alkalosis and to alkalinize urine.

Side and Adverse Effects. Common side effects associated with this agent are paresthesias of the tongue, lips, anus, and extremities and drowsiness. Other effects include hypokalemia and hypersensitivity reactions.

Contraindications and Cautions. This agent should not be used in individuals who are allergic to sulfonamides. It should be used cautiously in individuals with renal dysfunction and those taking digitalis.

NURSING IMPLICATIONS

• May be taken with food to minimize possibility of gastrointestinal upset.
• Diuretic dose is generally administered in the morning to avoid nocturia.

$$CO_2 + H_2O \xrightarrow{\text{carbonic anhydrase}} H_2CO_3 \rightleftharpoons H^+ + HCO_3^-$$

Figure 10–7. The process by which carbon dioxide (CO_2) is hydrated by the enzyme carbonic anhydrase to form bicarbonate.

- Monitor intake and output when drug is used to reduce edema.
- Daily weights are advised as a useful index of response to diuretic action.
- Adequate fluid intake should be maintained during drug therapy to reduce risk of kidney stone formation due to the high alkalinity (approximately pH 9.2) of the drug.
- May cause substantial increases in blood glucose in diabetics and in pre-diabetics. Changes in drug dose or diet may be indicated.
- Monitor serum and urine electrolytes during therapy; especially advise the patient to report signs of hypokalemia and metabolic acidosis.

THIAZIDE DIURETICS

Action and Fate. The agents classified as thiazide diuretics are among the most commonly used diuretics (refer to Table 10–18 for individual agents). Chemically they are related to the sulfonamides. They produce diuresis by reducing sodium reabsorption, primarily in the kidney nephron at the distal portion of the loop of Henle (Fig. 10–6). Increased sodium excretion also leads to increased potassium excretion and bicarbonate excretion, and decreases calcium and uric acid excretion. The mechanism by which these agents lower elevated blood pressure is thought to be due in part to a vasodilation.

The thiazides are generally excreted unchanged in the urine. They cross the placenta and appear in breast milk.

Uses. The thiazide diuretics are Step 1 agents (refer to section on Antihypertensive Agents in this chapter), used alone or in conjunction with other antihypertensive agents in the management of hypertension. They are also used to treat edema associated with CHF, hepatic cirrhosis, renal dysfunction, corticosteroid or estrogen therapy.

Side and Adverse Effects. Electrolyte imbalance including hypokalemia, hypomagnesemia, and hyponatremia can occur with thiazide diuretics. They also cause hyperuricemia, hyperglycemia, and hyperlipidemia. Other side effects include hypersensitivity reactions.

Contraindications and Cautions. The use of thiazide and thiazide-like diuretics is contraindicated in individuals with known hypersensitivity reactions to sulfonamides. These agents are not effective diuretics in individuals with decreased glomerular filtration rate. They should be used cautiously in individuals with diabetes or gout.

NURSING IMPLICATIONS

- Administer diuretic in the morning to avoid nocturia. Best to administer after eating to prevent gastric irritations.

TABLE 10–18. THIAZIDE DIURETICS

Class of Diuretic	Site of Action	% Sodium Reabsorption Inhibited
Thiazide and thiazide-like diuretics	Ascending loop of Henle (cortical)	6–8
Loop diuretics	Ascending loop of Henle (medullary and possibly cortical)	20–25
Potassium-sparing diuretics	Distal tubule	2

- Monitor serum and urine electrolytes. Be alert for signs of hypokalemia (muscle cramps, weakness, mental confusion) and hyponatremia. Report these signs to physician.
- Baseline and periodic determinations of serum electrolytes, CBCs, blood urea nitrogen (BUN), blood glucose, uric acid, and CO_2 are recommended.
- May cause photosensitivity; advise patient to avoid direct sunlight and to use a sunscreen.
- Daily weights are recommended. Report sudden weight gain or loss.
- Monitor intake and output ratio.
- Thiazide therapy can cause hyperglycemia and glycosuria in diabetic and diabetic-prone individuals.
- Blood pressure should be monitored closely during early therapy.
- In patients with orthostatic hypertension, teach patient to change positions very slowly and in stages.
- Thiazide therapy can cause hyperuricemia, which precipitates gout.
- Potassium supplement or increased potassium-rich foods may be needed.

LOOP DIURETICS

Action and Fate. The loop diuretics (Table 10–16) act mainly by inhibiting sodium reabsorption along the ascending loop of Henle. To a lesser extent they also inhibit the reabsorption of sodium in the proximal and distal renal tubules of the nephrons.

These agents are metabolized in the liver and excreted for the most part in the urine. Only furosemide is primarily excreted unchanged. Furosemide crosses the placenta and appears in breast milk.

Uses. These potent diuretics are used to treat edema associated with CHF, liver or renal disease. Furosemide may be used instead of a thiazide diuretic in the management of hypertension in those individuals with decreased glomerular filtration rate.

Side and Adverse Effects. These agents can cause fluid and electrolyte imbalances such as hypovolemia, dehydration, hyponatremia, and hypokalemia. Postural hypotension may also occur. All three agents are associated with various types of ototoxicity. All three agents are also associated with hyperglycemia.

Contraindications and Cautions. Furosemides and bumetamide should not be given to individuals with known hypersensitivity reaction to sulfonamides. These agents should not be used in individuals with oliguria, anuria, hypovolemia, or electrolyte imbalances. Safe use of these agents during pregnancy has not been established.

NURSING IMPLICATIONS

- Schedule doses in AM to avoid nocturia.
- Periodic checks should be made of blood count, serum and electrolytes, CO_2, BUN, blood sugar, and uric acid.
- Monitor input–output ratio. Report decrease in output or excessive diuresis.
- Weigh patient daily; report rapid or excessive weight loss (from vigorous diuresis), which can induce dehydration and acute hypotensive episodes, especially in the elderly.
- Monitor blood pressure during periods of diuresis and through period of dosage adjustment.

- Patients receiving high doses are subject to episodes of postural hypotension usually experienced as lightheadedness, dizziness, weakness, and lethargy. Caution patient to change positions slowly, especially from a sitting to standing position.
- Be alert to signs of ototoxicity (hearing loss and tinnitus) when administering in conjunction with other ototoxic drugs.
- Acute gout can occur in susceptible patients. Advise patient to report onset of joint redness, swelling, or pain.
- Check with physician on allowable salt and fluid intake. Also may need to increase intake of potassium-rich foods, or a potassium supplement may be needed.

POTASSIUM-SPARING DIURETICS

Action and Fate. This class of diuretics consists of two unrelated agents. Spirono-lactone is a steroid compound which blocks aldosterone receptors in the distal renal tubule. It is rapidly metabolized in the liver and the metabolites excreted in the urine. It crosses the placenta.

Triamterene enhances sodium excretion by direct action at the distal tubule. It is metabolized in the liver and excreted in the urine.

Both agents promote sodium excretion without potassium loss.

Uses. Both agents have weak diuretic action. Spironolactone is used in conditions such as hypertension, edema due to CHF, hepatic cirrhosis, and nephrotic syndrome associated with an increased production of aldosterone and with potassium-depleting agents to reduce potassium loss (available with hydrochloro-thiazide as Aldactazide).

The use of triamterene is indicated for the same conditions as spironolactone. It is most often combined with potassium-depleting agents to reduce potassium loss (available with hydrochlorothiazide as Dyazide and Maxzide).

Side and Adverse Effects. Both agents can produce fluid and electrolyte imbalance consisting of hyponatremia and hyperkalemia. Both agents can cause lethargy, confusion, fatigue, and headache. Spironalactone may cause gynecomastia in men and virilizing effects in women.

Contraindications and Cautions. These agents should be used carefully in individuals with electrolyte imbalances, especially hyperkalemia and hyponatremia, anuria, and renal insufficiency.

NURSING IMPLICATIONS

- Schedule doses in AM to prevent nocturia.
- Periodic checks should be made on blood counts, BUN, serum creatinine and serum potassium levels.
- Observe for signs and symptoms of hyperkalemia, unusual fatigue, weakness or heaviness of limbs, general muscle weakness, muscle cramps and paresthesias, shortness of breath, nervousness, confusion, and cardiac arrhythmias as these drugs promote potassium retention.
- Monitor daily intake and output and check for edema. Report lack of diuretic response or development of edema to physician.
- Weigh patient prior to therapy for baseline information and throughout therapy.
- Gynecomastia may appear in males with spironolactone, but may be related to dosage level and duration of therapy. It may persist in some patients even after drug is stopped.

Calcium Channel Blockers

Until only recently, myocardial infarct and angina pectoris were thought to be caused solely by atherosclerosis. New technology in coronary arteriography has made it possible to observe the heart in action and to see otherwise normal coronary arteries undergoing spasm. This spasm can disrupt blood flow as effectively as atherosclerosis and can lead to either a myocardial infarct or angina pectoris. This type of angina is known as vasospastic or Prinzmetal's angina. Management of this type of angina is with a new class of agents known as the calcium channel blockers. Currently there are three calcium channel blockers available: diltiazem (Cardizem), nifedipine (Procardia), and verapamil (Calan, Isoptin).

Action and Fate. Even though all three agents are structurally dissimilar, they do share a common mechanism of action. They inhibit the passage of calcium ions into muscle cells through specific channels known as slow channels. The exact means by which these agents accomplish this is not known. (Refer to Table 10–19 for other actions.)

   All three agents are metabolized in the liver. Diltiazem and verapamil are metabolized to active metabolites, nifedipine is not.

Uses. All three agents are indicated for use in vasospastic or Prinzmetal's angina and stable angina. Verapamil is also indicated in the treatment of supraventricular tachyarrhythmias.

Side and Adverse Effects. Refer to Table 10–20 for side and adverse effects.

Contraindications and Cautions. Sick sinus syndrome (unless functional pacemaker is in place), second or third degree AV block, hepatic and renal dysfunction. Cautious use in CHF. Verapamil should not be used simultaneously with beta blockers.

NURSING IMPLICATIONS

- May cause transient hypotension; monitor blood pressure closely.
- If given concurrently with a digitalis preparation, monitor closely for heart block.
- Hold medication if pulse is irregular or slower than base level.
- Obtain heart rate and blood pressure prior to administration and withhold and call physician if hypotension or bradycardia are present.
- Contraindicated with beta blockers such as propanolol, as this may precipitate bradycardia.
- Instruct patient to change positions slowly to avoid pooling of blood.

TABLE 10–19. FREQUENCY OF VARIOUS CARDIOVASCULAR EFFECTS OF CALCIUM CHANNEL BLOCKERS

Generic Name	Trade Name	Effect			
		Coronary Vasodilation	Peripheral Vasodilation	Heart Rate	AV Conduction
diltiazem	Cardizem	+++	+	↓	↓
nifedipine	Procardia	+++	+++	↑	—
verapamil	Calan, Isoptin	++	++	↓↓	↑↓

+ = minimum effect; ++ = intermediate effect; +++ = maximum effect.

TABLE 10–20. FREQUENCY OF VARIOUS SIDE EFFECTS ATTRIBUTED TO THE CALCIUM CHANNEL BLOCKERS

Side Effects	diltiazem (%)	nifedipine (%)	verapamil (%)
Headache	2.0	23	1.8
Dizziness	—	27	3.6
Flushing	—	25	—
Weakness	—	12	—
Constipation	—	—	6.3
Hypotension	—	—	2.9
Nausea	2.7	—	—
Edema	2.4	—	—
Arrhythymias	2.0	—	—

Anticoagulants

The process by which blood clots in the body is an intricate and complex process. The coagulation scheme or cascade, as it is called, is shown in Figure 10–8. In addition to clotting factors the body also has anticlotting factors (Table 10–21). These substances act in conjunction with the clotting factors to prevent the formation of clots in blood vessels, and they also can dissolve small clots should they happen to form in blood vessels. When the normal balance between the clotting and anticlotting factors is disturbed for some reason, and depending on which factors predominate, the individual will experience either uncontrollable bleeding or clotting (thromboembolic) disorders. In the case of the thromboembolic disorders, an anticoagulant is used to prevent the formation of new clots; these agents do not dissolve any clots that are present. Heparin and warfarin are the mainstay of anticoagulant therapy. They both possess the same action, i.e.,

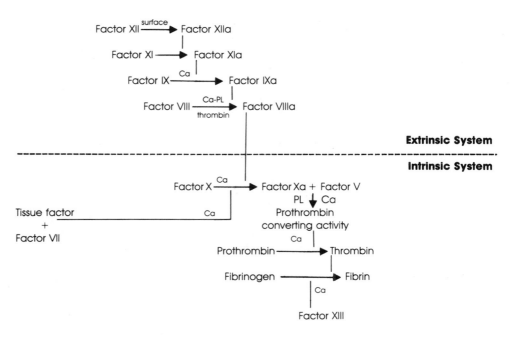

Figure 10–8. Mechanism of blood coagulation.

TABLE 10-21. BLOOD COAGULATION FACTORS

Factor	Other Designation
I	Fibrinogen
II	Prothrombin
III	Thromboplastin
IV	Calcium
V	Proaccelerin, plasma Ac-globulin, labile factor
VII	Proconvertin, stable factor, serum prothrombin conversion accelerator
VIII	Antihemophilic factor (AHF), antihemophilic factor A, antihemophilic globulin
IX	Plasma thromboplastin component (PTC), Christmas factor; antihemophilic factor B
X	Stuart–Prower factor
XI	Plasma thromboplastin antecedent (PTA), antihemophilic factor C
XII	Hageman factor, glass factor

the prevention of clot formation, but the mechanism by which they accomplish this differs (Table 10–22). Both agents are invaluable in the treatment of various cardiovascular diseases.

Heparin

Action and Fate. Heparin is a strongly acidic high molecular weight polysaccharide extracted from either bovine lung tissue or porcine intestinal mucosa. It prolongs the clotting of blood by preventing the formation of fibrin in the extrinsic system (Fig. 10–7) by inhibiting the actions of antithrombin III. This prevents the conversion of prothrombin to thrombin and thus the conversion of fibrinogen to fibrin. This action prolongs whole blood clotting time, thrombin time, partial thromboplastin time, and prothrombin time.

Heparin is metabolized in the liver and excreted by the kidneys both as unchanged drug and inactive metabolites.

Uses. Heparin is used to prevent the formation of venous thrombosis and pulmonary embolisms. It may be given either intravenously or subcutaneously. Intramuscular injection is not recommended. Additional uses for heparin include the prevention of thromboembolic complications associated with cardiac or vascular surgery and during the acute stage of a myocardial infarction. It may also be used prior to noncardiovascular surgery procedures, such as hysterectomies, as a prophylactic measure to prevent clot formation.

Heparin may also be used in the treatment of disseminated intravascular clotting syndrome (DIC) and as an anticoagulant in blood that is to be transfused and during dialysis procedures.

TABLE 10-22. COMPARISON OF HEPARIN AND WARFARIN

Generic Name	Trade Name	Onset of Action	Dura-tion	Route of Adminis-tration	Laboratory Control Tests	Overdose Treatment	Cost
heparin	—	Immediate IV: minutes SQ: 20–60 minutes	4 hr	Parenteral	Partial thrombo-plastin time (PTT)	Protamine sulfate	Expensive
warfarin	Coumadin Panwarfarin	Gradual, peaks in 48 hr	2–5 day	Oral and parenteral	Prothrombin time (PT)	Blood, plasma, or vitamin K	Inexpensive

Side and Adverse Effects. Individuals undergoing therapy with heparin can experience spontaneous bleeding, allergic reactions both local or systemic, and transient thrombocytopenia.

Contraindications and Cautions. Hypersensitivity reactions to heparin would preclude its use. Also, its use would be contraindicated in any individual with active bleeding or conditions that would predispose the individual to bleeding such as hemophilia, purpura, or thrombocytopenia. Heparin should be used cautiously in osteoporosis or during menstruation or pregnancy.

Warfarin

Action and Fate. Warfarin indirectly interferes with the blood clotting mechanism by depressing hepatic synthesis of vitamin K-dependent coagulation factors: factor II, prothrombin, factor VII, proconvertin, factor IX (Christmas factor), and factor X (Stuart–Prower factor). Warfarin has no effect on existing coagulation factors already circulating in the body. Warfarin has no effect on preformed clots; it does, however, prevent formation of new clots and limits the growth of existing clots.

Warfarin is metabolized in the liver and excreted in the urine and in the feces primarily as inactive metabolites.

Uses. Warfarin may be given orally, intramuscularly, or intravenously. The usual route is orally. Because of its delayed onset of action, it is used mainly as maintenance therapy to prevent the formation of deep venous thrombosis, pulmonary embolism, and in the treatment of atrial fibrillation with embolization. It is also used for the treatment of coronary occlusion, transient ischemic attacks, and in individuals with prosthetic heart valves.

Side and Adverse Effects. By far the major concern with warfarin is major or minor bleeding from any tissue or organ. In addition, anorexia, urticaria, purpura, and alopecia can occur.

Contraindications and Cautions. The use of warfarin is contraindicated in individuals with conditions that may cause bleeding, i.e., individuals with hemophilia, vitamin K deficiency, blood dyscrasias, and active peptic ulcer. Cautious use is indicated in women during menstruation, pregnancy, and while breast feeding.

Nursing Implications for Heparin and Warfarin

- Obtain prothrombin time (PT) (warfarin) partial thromboplastin time (PTT) (heparin), clotting times, platelets, hematocrit, and hemoglobin levels prior to admission for baseline information.
- PT and PTT levels must be obtained in AM if patient is on heparin for anticoagulation purposes. Call physician if PTT level is less than 2.5 times normal (indicates need for increased heparin) or greater than 3 times normal (indicates need for less heparin—patient is at risk of hemorrhaging).
- Monitor hematocrit and hemoglobin levels to indicate slow or acute hemorrhage.
- Protect from injury by padding side rails and assist patient in position changes.
- Prophylactic doses are administered subcutaneously in the abdominal area and injection sites rotated. Do not withdraw plunger to check entry into blood vessel. Do not rub or massage site; this will cause a subcutaneous hemorrhage and subsequent bruising.
- It is important to change the needle after drawing up heparin or the injection site will be heparinized and local hemorrhaging will occur.

- DO NOT DISCONTINUE drug abruptly. Heparin usage must be weaned to oral warfarin dosage.
- Observe for and report signs and symptoms of excessive bleeding, such as: increased heart rate with decreased blood pressure, nosebleeds, tarry stools, or increased menstrual flow. Test urine, stool, and emesis for occult blood.
- Use soft bristle toothbrush to prevent bleeding gums; an electric razor is recommended for shaving.
- Advise patient not to use aspirin or aspirin-containing medications.
- Antidote for heparin overdose is protamine sulfate and the antidote for warfarin overdose is vitamin K.

Review Questions

CARDIAC GLYCOSIDES

The two drugs usually used to treat congestive heart failure are digoxin and digitoxin. Give two reasons why digoxin is preferred over digitoxin.

1. _____

2. _____

3. Which two of the following four drugs interfere with the excretion of digoxin?

   propranolol
   quinidine
   furosemide
   calcium channel blockers

   a. propranolol and quinidine
   b. propranolol and calcium channel blockers
   c. quinidine and calcium channel blockers
   d. propranolol and furosemide

4. Define what is meant by the term digitalizing dose.

5. Which of the following factors may cause an increase in digoxin serum concentration?
   a. renal failure
   b. quinidine administration
   c. administration of a calcium channel blocker
   d. all of the above

6. All of the following may be associated with digitalis toxicity EXCEPT:
   a. nausea, anorexia
   b. fatigue, confusion
   c. acute renal failure
   d. apical pulse below 60

7. Digoxin exerts its pharmacological effect by exerting a:
   a. positive inotropy and negative chronotropy
   b. negative inotropy and positive chronotropy
   c. negative inotropy and negative chronotropy
   d. none of the above

8. The therapeutic blood level for digoxin (Lanoxin) is:
   a. 0.8 to 2.0 Gm/ml
   b. 0.8 to 2.0 mcg/ml

     c. 0.8 to 2.0 ng/ml
     d. 0.8 to 2.0 mg/ml

9. Which digitalis preparation has the longest half-life ($t_{1/2}$)?
    a. digoxin
    b. digitoxin

ANTIARRHYTHMIA AGENTS

10. A lupus-like syndrome has been associated with the use of which drug?
    a. lidocaine
    b. atropine
    c. procainamide
    d. bretylium

11. The initial dose of which one of the following antiarrhythmic drugs is given as a bolus of 50 to 100 mg (1 mg/kg)?
    a. lidocaine
    b. phenytoin
    c. procainamide
    d. quinidine

12. Quinidine will produce in sensitive individuals certain symptoms known as "cinchonism." These symptoms include:
    a. rash, fever, arthritis
    b. nausea, vomiting, diarrhea
    c. tinnitus, headache, disturbed vision
    d. bradycardia, anorexia, gynecomastia

13. You should closely observe a patient taking Pronestyl (procainamide) for which of the following?
    a. joint pains, rash
    b. bradycardia, hypotension
    c. tachycardia, hypertension
    d. dystonias, Parkinson-like symptoms

14. The drug of choice for digoxin-induced heart arrhythmias is:
    a. Pronestyl
    b. lidocaine
    c. quinidine
    d. Dilantin

15. Electrical impulses of the heart normally originate from the:
    a. sinus (SA) node
    b. atrioventricular (AV) node
    c. ventricular cells
    d. right atrium

16–23. Matching:

Generic Name	Trade Name
16. _____ disopyramide	a. Calan, Isoptin
17. _____ phenytoin	b. Procan-SR, Pronestyl
18. _____ acebutolol	c. Tonocard
19. _____ bretylium	d. Dilantin
20. _____ verapamil	e. Norpace
21. _____ procainamide	f. Bretylol
22. _____ tocainide	g. Sectral
23. _____ propranolol	h. Inderal

ANTIANGINAL AGENTS

Give the three classes of drugs used to treat angina.

24. *Nitrates*

25. *Beta Blockers*

26. *Ca++ Channel Blockers*   p, 195

27. Give the mechanism of action by which nitrates alleviate an anginal attack.

28. Nitrates are available as:
    a. sublingual tablets
    b. transdermal patches
    c. a sublingual metered aerosol
    d. all of the above

29. Nitrates should be used cautiously in patients with which of the following:

    renal dysfunction
    hepatic dysfunction
    early myocardial infarct
    emphysema

    The correct answers are:

    a. renal dysfunction, hepatic dysfunction, and emphysema
    b. renal dysfunction and hepatic dysfunction
    c. hepatic dysfunction and early myocardial infarct
    d. renal dysfunction, hepatic dysfunction, early myocardial infarct, and emphysema

30. Common side effects associated with sublingual nitroglycerin tablets include:
    a. headache
    b. syncope
    c. postural hypotension
    d. all of the above

31. IV solutions of nitroglycerin must be:
    a. protected from light
    b. mixed in a glass bottle
    c. filtered during administration
    d. mixed in lactated Ringer's

32. The oral long-acting nitrites are used prophylactically for angina. Theoretically these drugs should not be effective because they are:
    a. destroyed by gastric acid
    b. not lipid soluble therefore not absorbed
    c. susceptible to the first pass effect
    d. destroyed by the basic pH in the gut

33. Prinzmetal's angina, which is a variant type, is most effectively controlled with:
    a. nitrites
    b. propranolol
    c. nitroglycerin IV
    d. calcium channel blockers

Explain why it is important to instruct the patient to:

34. sit or lie down prior to taking nitroglycerin tablets sublingually.

35. keep sublingual tablets in the original amber glass container.

36. discard sublingual tablets and obtain a new supply 6 months after opening the bottle.

ANTIHYPERTENSIVE AGENTS

37. Blood pressure must be in excess of _____ recorded at _____ separate times in order to be defined as hypertension.

If hypertension is left untreated or left inadequately treated, damage will occur to what four organ systems?

38. _____

39. _____

40. _____

41. _____

List the three beta blockers that have cardioselective action.

42. _____

43. _____

44. _____

45–51. Matching:

Drug	Side Effect
45. __B__ methyldopa	a. bronchospasm
46. __E__ reserpine	b. high incidence of sexual dysfunction
47. ____ hydralazine	c. reflex tachycardia
48. __A__ propranolol	d. first dose phenomenon
49. ____ prazosin	e. severe depression
50. ____ minoxidil	f. hypertrichosis
51. ____ captopril	g. ageusia

52. Which of the following is a possible long-term consequence of poorly controlled hypertension?
    a. strokes
    b. renal failure
    c. congestive heart failure
    d. all of the above

53. A beta blocker is commonly given with hydralazine for hypertension because:
    a. the beta blocker inhibits hydralazine-induced tachycardia
    b. hydralazine inhibits beta blocker-induced bronchospasm
    c. neither drug has central nervous system side effects
    d. none of the above

54. Which beta blocker is available for topical use in glaucoma?
    a. timolol
    b. propranolol
    c. metoprolol
    d. nadolol

55. Abrupt withdrawal of beta blockers has resulted in:
    a. a decrease in anginal symptoms
    b. hypertension
    c. strokes
    d. myocardial infarct

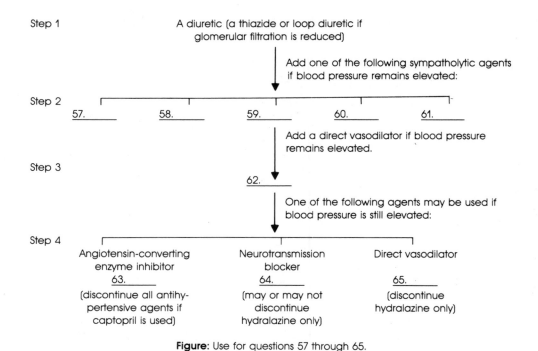

Step 1   A diuretic (a thiazide or loop diuretic if glomerular filtration is reduced)

Add one of the following sympatholytic agents if blood pressure remains elevated:

Step 2   57.____   58.____   59.____   60.____   61.____

Add a direct vasodilator if blood pressure remains elevated.

Step 3   62.____

One of the following agents may be used if blood pressure is still elevated:

Step 4

| Angiotensin-converting enzyme inhibitor 63.____ (discontinue all antihypertensive agents if captopril is used) | Neurotransmission blocker 64.____ (may or may not discontinue hydralazine only) | Direct vasodilator 65.____ (discontinue hydralazine only) |

Figure: Use for questions 57 through 65.

56. Propranolol has been approved to treat hypertension, angina pectoris, cardiac arrhythmias, and:
    a. migraine headaches
    b. myasthenia gravis
    c. Cushing's syndrome
    d. Addison's disease

57.–65. Fill in the blanks in the figure above with the correct drug name (generic and trade).

DIURETICS

66–76. Identify the correct location of the following in the figure on the next page.

66. Bowman's capsule   _____
67. glomerulus   _____
68. loop of Henle   _____
69. proximal tubule   _____
70. distal tubule   _____
71. descending limb   _____
72. ascending limb   _____
73. collecting duct   _____
74. site of action of thiazides   _____
75. site of action for loop diuretics   _____
76. site of action for potassium-sparing diuretics   _____

Give the three basic ways in which diuretics act.

77. _____

78. _____

79. _____

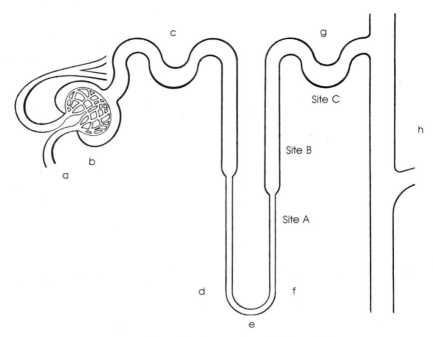

Figure: Use for questions 66 through 76.

Give the five classes of diuretics.

80. _____

81. _____

82. _____

83. _____

84. _____

85. Furosemide is a _____ diuretic.
    a. potassium-sparing
    b. potassium-depleting

86–92. Matching:

Drug	**Class**
86. _____ mannitol	a. loop diuretic
87. _____ urea	b. thiazide diuretic
88. _____ acetazolamide	c. osmotic diuretic
89. _____ hydrochlorothiazide	d. potassium-sparing diuretic
90. _____ spironolactone	e. carbonic anhydrase inhibitor
91. _____ triamterene	
92. _____ furosemide	

93–101. Matching:

Trade Name	**Generic Name**
93. _____ HydroDiuril	a. spironolactone
94. _____ Aldactone	b. chlorothiazide
95. _____ Osmitrol	c. furosemide
96. _____ Dyazide	d. hydrochlorothiazide
97. _____ Diuril	e. mannitol
98. _____ Esidrex	f. triamterene/hydrochlorothiazide
99. _____ Lasix	g. acetazolamide
100. _____ Oretic	
101. _____ Diamox	

102–106. Match the agent with the side effect:

Agent	Side Effect
102. _____ furosemide	a. dry mouth, excessive diuresis, headache
103. _____ mannitol	b. paresthesias of the tongue, lips, anus, and extremities
104. _____ spironolactone	c. hypokalemia, hyperglycemia, hyperuricemia
105. _____ thiazide diuretics	d. hyperkalemia, gynecomastia in men, virilizing effects in women
106. _____ acetazolamide	e. hypokalemia, ototoxicity

107. An individual taking a thiazide diuretic for hypertension complains of leg cramps for 2 weeks after therapy is initiated. This would most likely be due to:
   a. a decreased serum sodium level
   b. a decreased serum potassium level
   c. an increased uric acid level
   d. an elevated blood glucose level

CALCIUM CHANNEL BLOCKERS

108. The calcium channel blocker with the highest incidence of side effects is _____.

109. All three calcium channel blockers are indicated for use in:
   a. supraventricular tachycardia
   b. vasospastic angina
   c. congestive heart failure
   d. hypotension

110–113. Matching:

Trade Name	Generic Name
110. _b_ Procardia	a. diltiazem
111. _c_ Isoptin	b. nifedipine
112. _a_ Cardizem	c. verapamil
113. _c_ Calan	

ANTICOAGULANTS

114. Protamine sulfate is given:
   a. PO to neutralize heparin overdose
   b. IV to neutralize heparin overdose
   c. IM for minor bleeding
   d. IV to neutralize warfarin overdose

115. The laboratory test of choice for monitoring heparin therapy is:
   a. prothrombin time
   b. partial thromboplastin time
   c. bleeding time
   d. Lee and White clotting time

116. The laboratory test of choice for monitoring warfarin therapy is:
    a. prothrombin time
    b. partial thromboplastin time
    c. bleeding time
    d. Lee and White blood-clotting time

117. Which of the following is true regarding heparin administration?
    a. IM administration is used when prolonged therapy is indicated.
    b. SQ administration site may be either the iliac *or* the abdominal area.
    c. When administering subcutaneously, withdraw the plunger to make sure not to insert in a vein.
    d. When administering heparin, either IM or SQ, the area should be massaged for 5 to 10 seconds.

=11=

Adrenal Corticosteroids

The adrenal corticosteroids found in the body can be classed into two types: the glucocorticosteroids (cortisol [hydrocortisone], cortisone, and corticosterone) and the mineralocorticosteroids (aldosterone) (Table 11–1).

Both classes of hormones are synthesized in and subsequently released into the bloodstream by the adrenal cortex. Their release is controlled by the hypothalamus, which when stimulated by such factors as stress, trauma, and diurnal rhythms releases corticotropin releasing factor (CRF), which in turn signals the pituitary gland to release the adrenocorticotropic hormone (ACTH). ACTH then stimulates the release of the adrenal corticosteroids from the adrenal cortex. A negative feedback system regulates the production of these substances and, as the blood level of the adrenal corticosteroids rises, the release of CRF and ACTH is suppressed (Fig. 11–1).

There are numerous preparations, both natural and synthetic, available. They come in a variety of dose forms and have widespread applications. Efforts have been made in the development of the synthetic products to retain and even increase the beneficial effects of these agents and to diminish the undesirable side effects. Table 11–2 shows some of the more commonly encountered agents comparing their anti-inflammatory and sodium retention potentials.

Action and Fate. The corticosteroids must cross the cell membrane to be effective. Their action depends on complexing with their receptors that are located in the cytoplasm of cells and then this complex is transported into the cell nucleus. Once in the nucleus the receptor–steroid complex interacts with the DNA in such a way as to promote or "turn on" the synthesis of specific messenger RNAs that direct the synthesis of certain proteins (Fig. 11–2). In their normal physiological levels, glucocorticosteroids will regulate glucose metabolism by increasing liver glycogen stores and gluconeogenesis. They also are involved in lipid metabolism by promoting lipolysis and protein metabolism by supporting normal maintenance and function of skeletal muscles. In elevated blood levels, which occur when these agents are administered in pharmacological doses, an exaggeration of their normal functions occurs in addition to other effects such as anti-inflammatory, antiallergic actions; suppression of the immune system; suppression of normal growth in children; and mood and psychic alterations.

The mineralocorticosteroids in physiological amounts act at the distal renal tubules to regulate sodium retention and potassium loss. At pharmacological levels, their action is essentially the same, only the intensity of their effect differs.

The adrenal corticosteroids are metabolized in the liver for the most part into water-soluble substances and then excreted by the kidneys via the urine. Two adrenal corticosteroids, cortisone and prednisone, must be metabolized to active products (hydrocortisone and prednisolone, respectively) before they are pharmacologically active.

111

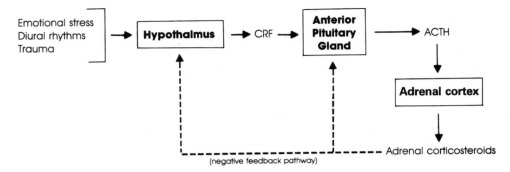

Figure 11–1. Schematic representation of the hypothalamus-pituitary-adrenal (HPA) axis showing the release of corticotropin-releasing factor (CRF), the subsequent release of adrenocorticotropic hormone (ACTH), and finally the release of corticosteroids by the adrenal cortex. As the circulating level of steroids increases, the release of CRF and ACTH is suppressed by the negative feedback pathway.

Uses. Uses of these agents are numerous. In combination, i.e., a glucocortocosteroid and a mineralocorticosteroid, they are used as replacement therapy in the treatment of acute or chronic adrenal insufficiency (Addison's disease).

The majority of uses, however, involve the glucocorticosteroids alone. These agents are used in those situations or conditions requiring the intervention of an allergic response or suppression of the immune system. Some of the conditions for which these agents are used include asthma, renal disease, collagen diseases, rheumatic endocarditis, certain ocular disorders, ulcerative colitis, skin diseases, severe allergic reactions, and organ transplants. They are not considered an initial choice in the treatment of arthritis, but are considered when nonsteroidal anti-inflammatory agents have failed. In these cases, they may be injected directly into the affected joint, intra-articularly, or given by the oral route. Specific glucocorticosteroids have specific uses. One is dexamethasone, which is used to reduce cerebral edema and to reverse the detrimental effects of septic shock. The other agent is prednisone, which is also used for septic shock and in certain chemotherapeutic protocols. (The use of corticosteroids in the treatment of cancer is discussed in Chapter 17.)

Side and Adverse Effects. Adrenal corticosteroids can cause a wide range of side and adverse effects, with the glucocorticosteroids causing the most serious ones. Pharmacological doses of either type of corticosteroids taken for more than 5 to 10 days will lead to the suppression of adrenal synthesis of these hormones. For this reason, agents taken under these circumstances must be tapered off and not abruptly discontinued. (See Principles of Administration under Nursing Implica-

TABLE 11–1. SOME GLUCOCORTICOSTEROIDS AND MINERALOCORTICOSTEROIDS

Generic Name	Trade Name
Glucocorticosteroids	
cortisone (naturally occurring)	Cortone
hydrocortisone (naturally occurring)	—
betamethasone	Celestone
dexamethasone	Decadron, Hexadrol
prednisolone	Delta-Cortef, Orasone
prednisone	Deltasone
triamcinolone	Aristocort, Kenalog
Mineralocorticosteroids	
aldosterone (naturally occurring)	—
desoxycorticosterone	DOCA
fludrocortisone	Florinef

TABLE 11–2. THE ANTI-INFLAMMATORY POTENCY, EQUIVALENT ORAL DOSES, AND POTENTIAL FOR SODIUM RETENTION[a]

Generic Name	Trade Name	Anti-Inflammatory Potency	Equivalent Oral Dose (mg)	Sodium Retention Potential
hydrocortisone	—	1.0	20	2+
cortisone	Cortone	0.8	25	2+
prednisolone	Delta-Cortef Orasone	5.0	5	1+
prednisone	Deltasone	4.0	5	1+
methylprednisolone	Medrol	5.0	4	0
triamcinolone	Aristocort Kenalog	5.0	4	0
betamethasone	Celestone	40.0	0.6	0
dexamethasone	Decadron Hexadrol	30.0	0.75	0

[a] For commonly used glucocorticosteroids, using hydrocortisone as the base of comparison.

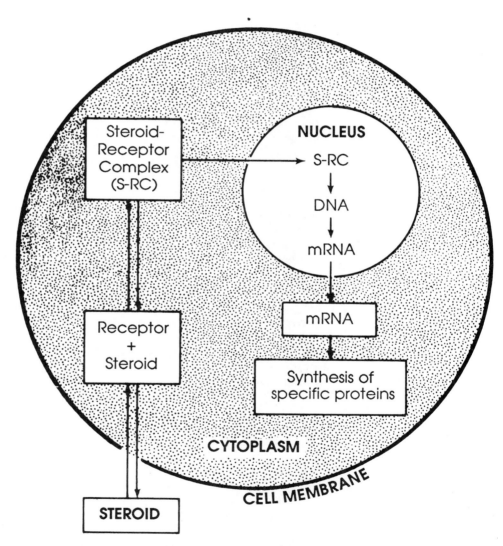

Figure 11–2. Steps in the action of adrenal corticosteroids. The steroid must penetrate the cell membrane and complex with its receptor, which is located in the cytoplasm, the S-RC. This complex, then, enables the steroid to enter the cell nucleus where it directs the DNA to synthesize specific messenger RNA (mRNA). This mRNA then directs the synthesis of specific proteins in the cytoplasm. The synthesis of these proteins is responsible for the effects of adrenal corticosteroids on the body. (*Adapted from Katzung BG (ed): Basic and Clinical Pharmacology, 3rd ed. East Norwalk, Conn, Appleton & Lange, 1987, with permission.*)

TABLE 11-3. SUMMARY OF COMPLICATIONS THAT CAN ACCOMPANY LONG-TERM THERAPY WITH ADRENAL CORTICOSTEROIDS

Musculoskeletal
Myopathy
Osteoporosis
Growth retardation in children

Gastrointestinal
Peptic ulceration with bleeding and ulceration
Gastric blood loss

Central Nervous System
Mood changes
Psychiatric disorders ("steroid psychosis")

Ophthalmologic
Glaucoma
Posterior subcapsular cataracts

Cardiovascular and Renal
Hypertension
Edema related to sodium retention
Precipitation or worsening of congestive heart failure
Hypokalemia

Metabolic
Precipitation or worsening of diabetes
Hyperlipidemia
Weight gain

Endocrine
Secondary amenorrhea
Suppression of adrenal gland synthesis of steroids

Suppression of Immune Response
Increased susceptibility to infections including bacterial, fungal, and viral

Inhibition of Fibroblastic Function
Poor wound healing

Induction of Cushing's Syndrome
Physical alterations in the body, which include thickening of the trunk, deposition of fat on upper back ("buffalo hump"), rounding of the face ("moon face"), thinning of the extremities

tions.) The prolonged use of glucocorticosteroids is associated with the development of a Cushing-like syndrome. Changes in the individual physically include a rounding of the face also known as a "moon face," redistribution of body fat to the trunk making it thicker, a decrease of muscle mass of the extremities making them thin, and the deposition of fat on the upper back causing the formation of a hump also known as a "buffalo hump." The other side effects are listed in Table 11–3. Keep in mind that the glucocorticosteroids that do not possess mineralocorticosteroid properties are less likely to cause the side effects associated with sodium and fluid retention such as hypertension, edema, and potassium depletion.

The side effects of the mineralocorticosteroids are not as extensive; they are more of an intensification of their normal physiological effects. These include, in addition to adrenal suppression, hypertension and sodium retention, which lead to edema, hypokalemia, and headache.

Contraindications and Cautions. Conditions that would warrant careful administration of these agents with close monitoring of the patient would include individuals with diabetes or a family history of diabetes, those diagnosed as having a psychosis, and those with or having a history of peptic ulcers. These agents should be used cautiously in those with glaucoma and cardiovascular diseases. These agents should not be used in those individuals who have viral or bacterial infections, tuberculosis, or Cushing's syndrome, unless their therapeutic advantage outweighs the risk.

NURSING IMPLICATIONS

- Principles of rational administration of corticosteroids:

    When possible, the administration of corticosteroids should mimic the natural secretion of these hormones. Peak secretion of corticosteroids occurs (for those on normal work schedules) at about 2 AM to 8 AM. Therefore it is best to give these medications at 8 AM to minimize the adrenal suppression.

    If less than 25 mg of prednisone per day is given or the equivalent, and the medication taken at 8 AM for fewer than 5 to 10 days, there is usually no adrenal suppression.

    Any deviation from this dosing regimen will suppress adrenal function. Once the medication is discontinued, the hypothalamus-pituitary-adrenal (HPA) axis will not respond appropriately to stressful situations. This can be fatal for the individual. For this reason the individual should be tapered off the medication.

Once the HPA axis is suppressed, it may take up to 1 year for full normal function to return. It is therefore advisable to ascertain prior to any surgical procedure if the individual has taken steroids during the past year. If so they will require a dose of hydrocortisone to help cope with the stress induced by the surgical procedure. The same is true for individuals with severe infections.

When giving steroids to children, an alternate day therapy regimen is advisable in order to minimize growth suppression.

- Do not confuse adrenal corticosteroids with the anabolic steroids used by individuals to increase muscle mass.
- Glucocorticosteroids may be administered with antacids to minimize the dyspepsia associated with them.
- Observe and note changes in patient's behavior. Watch for euphoria, depression, paranoia ("steroid psychosis").
- Monitor patient for edema and alterations in blood pressure, even if there is no history of cardiovascular disease.
- Monitor patient closely for complaints that could indicate alterations in glucose metabolism (hyperglycemia). If the patient is a known diabetic, alterations in the medication dose may be needed.
- For individuals with liver disease, the active form of prednisone (prednisolone) should be used.

Review Questions

1. The major function of the mineralocorticosteroids is to maintain the proper balance of fluid electrolytes. When a decrease in plasma volume occurs, the adrenal gland will begin to secrete these hormones in order to:
   a. deplete sodium
   b. retain sodium
   c. retain potassium
   d. none of the above

2. A deficiency of corticosteroids is characterized by hyperpigmentation, weakness, and hypotension. This is known as:
   a. Cushing's syndrome
   b. Addison's disease
   c. Crohn's disease
   d. lupus

3. For those children who have asthma and must be treated with steroids, it is desirable to dose them on an every other day schedule because daily dosing can cause:
   a. congestive heart failure
   b. a decrease in the number of circulating granulocytes
   c. inhibition of normal bone growth
   d. none of the above

4. The use of glucocorticosteroids is contraindicated and must be evaluated in terms of risk versus benefit for those patients who have:
   a. peptic ulcer
   b. peptic ulcer and psychosis
   c. peptic ulcer, psychosis, and tuberculosis
   d. peptic ulcer, psychosis, tuberculosis, and arthritis

5. Abrupt discontinuation of steroids after long-term use can lead to a life-threatening situation because:
   a. rebound hypertension will occur
   b. hypotension will occur

    c. the patient will become susceptible to infection

    d. adrenal suppression has occurred

6. If a patient is taking digoxin daily for congestive heart failure, would treating them with a glucocorticosteroid for a prolonged period of time be contraindicated?

    a. yes

    b. no

7–11. Matching:

Steroid	**Type**
7. ___hydrocortisone	a. glucocorticoid
8. ___fludrocortisone	b. mineralocorticoid
9. ___cortisone	
10. ___aldosterone	
11. ___desoxycorticosterone	

12. Prednisolone should be used in those patients who also have:

    a. congestive heart failure

    b. decreased renal function

    c. cirrhosis

    d. lupus

13. The recommended dosing time for steroids, based on the normal cycle of peak steroid release in the body, is:

    a. early in the morning

    b. late in the afternoon

    c. early evening

    d. late evening

14. When teaching the patient safe, self-administration of steroid therapy, which of the following would the nurse not include:

    a. the medication should not be stopped abruptly

    b. the medication should be taken with a meal or snack

    c. the patient should protect himself or herself from contracting infections

    d. all of the above

=12=

Sex Hormones and Related Agents

Female Hormones and Related Agents

ESTROGENS AND PROGESTINS

There are two types of female hormones: the estrogens and the progestins. In premenopausal women, the estrogens are synthesized and secreted by the ovary and the cortex of the adrenal gland. In postmenopausal women, the synthesis in the ovary declines and only the adrenal gland remains active in the synthesis of this hormone. During pregnancy, the synthesis of estrogens is transferred from the ovaries to the placenta. The naturally occurring estrogens that are the most significant are estradiol and estrone. Estrogens exert several important functions in the female. Estrogens are necessary in the development of secondary sex characteristics. They are also necessary for the maintenance of a normal menstrual cycle and stimulate the proliferation of the tissue that lines the endometrium. Estrogens are classed according to their structure: steroidal versus nonsteroidal. The naturally occurring hormones have a steroidal structure, i.e., their structure is basically the same as the corticosteroids. Some of these agents are not water soluble and hence cannot be given orally, therefore they must be administered parenterally. Some other estrogen preparations, even though they are steroidal in structure, are attached to certain substances that render them water soluble (the conjugated estrogens). Since these latter agents are water soluble, they may be given orally. The first agents that were available, however, were the nonwater-soluble agents and in order to provide agents that could be given orally, the nonsteroidal agents were developed.

The other type of female hormone, the progestins, are secreted by the corpus luteum, the adrenal cortex, and the placenta during pregnancy. The naturally occurring progestin is progesterone. The major effect of this hormone is seen primarily during the second half of the menstrual cycle. Progesterone causes certain changes to occur in the endometrium, preparing it for the implantation of the fertilized ovum. Progesterone is said to have a secretory effect on the endometrium, whereas estrogens have a proliferative effect. Figure 12–1 shows the level changes of the hormones during the menstrual cycle.

Estrogens and progestins are available in a variety of preparations: oral preparations, topical creams, and injectables.

Action and Fate. Estrogens and progestins act on specific target tissues where their receptors are located. These target tissues include the breast, the uterus, and the vagina. Their mechanism of action is similar to that of the cortico-

118

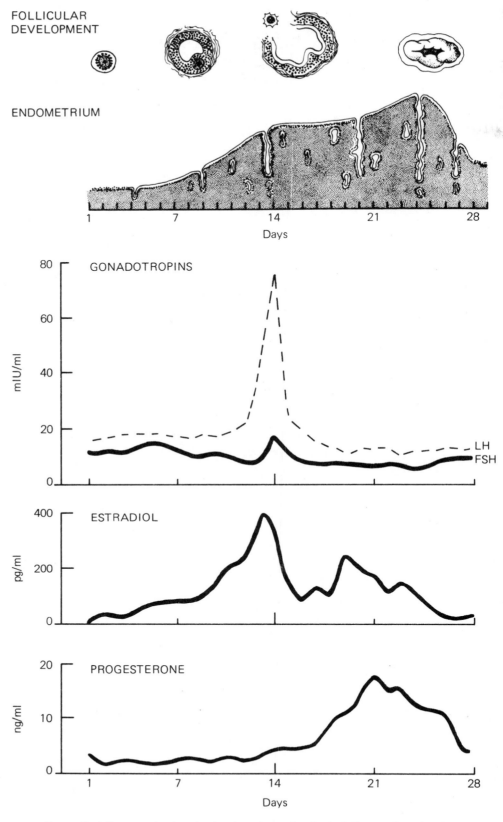

Figure 12–1. The menstrual cycle, showing plasma levels of pituitary and ovarian hormones and histological changes. (*From Katzung BG [ed]: Basic and Clinical Pharmacology, 2nd ed. Los Altos, Calif, Lange Medical Publications, 1984, with permission.*)

TABLE 12-1. COMMONLY USED ESTROGENS AND PROGESTINS

Generic Name	Trade Name	Route of Administration
Estrogens		
Steroidal		
estradiol	Estrace	PO
estrogens, conjugated	Premarin	PO, IM, IV, vaginal cream
estrogens, esterified	Estratab	PO
	Menest	
estropipate	Ogen	PO
ethinyl estradiol	Estinyl	PO, vaginal cream
quinestrol	Estrovis	PO
Nonsteroidal		
chlorotrianisene	Tace	PO
dienestrol	DES	PO, vaginal cream
diethylstilbestrol	Stilbestrol	vaginal cream or suppository
	OrthoDienestrol	
Progestins		
hydroxyprogesterone	Delalutin	IM
medroxyprogesterone	Amen	PO, IM
	Depo-Provera	
	Provera	
megestrol	Megace	PO

steroids. They must cross the cell membrane and enter the cytoplasm where they complex with their specific receptors. The receptor–hormone complex then enters the cell nucleus where the DNA is directed to synthesize specific messenger RNAs (mRNA), which in turn direct the synthesis of specific proteins.

Because most of these agents are highly lipid soluble, they must be metabolized in the liver before they can be excreted. Estrogens and progestins will cross the placenta and appear in breast milk.

Uses. Estrogens are used primarily to alleviate such vasomotor symptoms as hot flashes, dizziness, and sweating associated with natural or surgically induced menopause. They also retard the onset of osteoporosis, atrophy of the genitalia, pruritus vulvae, and vaginitis. Other situations where replacement therapy with estrogens is indicated are primary failure or inadequate function of the ovaries, prostatic cancer, and certain breast carcinomas. They are used in combination with a progestin in various formulations of oral contraceptives. Although not an approved use, diethylstilbestrol is used as an emergency postcoital contraceptive ("morning after") pill.

The progestins are used to treat secondary amenorrhea, functional uterine bleeding, endometriosis, and endometrial carcinoma. They may be used alone or in combination with an estrogen as oral contraceptives. They are also used in combination with an estrogen for treatment of menopausal symptoms.

Side and Adverse Effects. Some of the side effects seen with estrogens include fluid retention, nausea, vomiting, depression, increased size of uterine fibroid tumors, migraine headaches, increased levels of clotting factors, and precipitation of diabetes. In women still menstruating, break-through bleeding, dysmenorrhea, and amenorrhea may be experienced. Women who take estrogens to alleviate menopausal symptoms and who have not had their uterus removed run the increased risk of endometrial cancer.

The side effects of the progestins are essentially the same as the estrogens.

Contraindications and Cautions. The use of both hormones is contraindicated during pregnancy since they both have tetratogenic potential. Estrogens should not be used if an estrogen-dependent malignancy is present. If there is a history of hypertension, migraine headaches, or diabetes, both agents should be used with caution.

NURSING IMPLICATIONS

Estrogens

- To avoid overstimulation of target tissues and to mimic natural menses, estrogens are usually administered on a cyclic dosage regimen: 3 weeks on and 1 week off.
- In some cases, a progestational agent is added to the last 5 days of each cycle of estrogen therapy to produce more regularity.
- Behavioral changes or increasing mental depression may occur; if these symptoms persist, notify the physician.
- Reassure male patients that estrogen-induced feminization and impotence are reversible with termination of therapy.
- Advise diabetic users to report positive urine test promptly. Dosage adjustment of antidiabetic drug may be indicated.
- Regular yearly gynecologic check-ups (pap smears) and mammograms are advised for women using estrogen after menopause begins.
- Estrogen given intravenously should be infused very slowly to prevent flushing and tingling.

Progestins

- Progestins may cause some degree of fluid retention; also may cause some nausea.
- Inject deeply in administering agent IM. Do not rub injection site.
- Instruct a diabetic user of progestin to monitor clinical signs of loss of diabetes control. If urine tests become positive or hypoglycemic symptoms occur, the physician should be consulted.
- Yearly gynecologic check-ups are advised.

ORAL CONTRACEPTIVE AGENTS

The oral means of contraception was first introduced in the 1950s. The tablets usually contain a combination of both a synthetic estrogen and progestin derivative. This combination provides a convenient, reliable, and inexpensive means of birth control. A progestin alone can also be used as a birth control agent, but with less reliability.

Action and Fate. Birth control tablets that contain both an estrogenic agent and a progestational substance prevent ovulation by inhibiting the secretion of the gonadotropins, follicle-stimulating hormone, and luteinizing hormone, by the pituitary. Without them the follicles in the ovary do not develop and mature, and therefore release of the ovum or ovulation does not occur. Other changes that occur that also contribute to the contraceptive action of these agents include an increase in the viscosity of the cervical mucus, which makes it difficult for the sperm to penetrate the cervical opening, and tissue changes in the endometrium that prevent implantation of a fertilized ovum. The mechanism by which a progestin alone prevents conception is not fully understood, but probably involves increased viscosity of the cervical mucus and alterations in the endometrium.

The estrogens and progestins in birth control tablets are metabolized in the liver and excreted via the urine.

Uses. Birth control tablets are used to prevent pregnancy. Other uses include treatment of hypermenorrhea and endometriosis.

Side and Adverse Effects. The risks associated with birth control agents appear to increase with age (in individuals over 35) and in those who smoke. This is espe-

TABLE 12–2. VARIOUS BIRTH CONTROL PREPARATIONS

Trade Name	Estrogen	Progestin
Estrogen dominant		
Enovid E	mestranol 100 mcg	norethynodrel 2.5 mg
Norinyl 2 mg	mestranol 100 mcg	norethindrone 2 mg
Ortho-Novum 2 mg	mestranol 100 mcg	norethindrone 2 mg
Ovulen	mestranol 100 mcg	ethynodiol diacetate 1 mg
Intermediate		
Brevicon	ethinyl estradiol 35 mcg	norethindrone 0.5 mg
Demulen 1/50	ethinyl estradiol 50 mcg	ethynodiol diacetate 1 mg
Demulen 1/35	ethinyl estradiol 35 mcg	ethynodiol diacetate 1 mg
Enovid 5 mg	mestranol 75 mcg	norethynodrel 5 mg
Modicon	ethinyl estradiol 35 mcg	norethindrone 0.5 mg
Norinyl 1+80	mestranol 80 mcg	norethindrone 1 mg
Norinyl 1+50	mestranol 50 mcg	norethindrone 1 mg
Norlestrin 1/50	ethinyl estradiol 50 mcg	norethindrone 1 mg
Ortho-Novum 1/80	mestranol 80 mcg	norethindrone 1 mg
Ortho-Novum 1/50	mestranol 50 mcg	norethindrone 1 mg
Ortho-Novum 1/35	ethinyl estradiol 35 mcg	norethindrone 1 mg
Ortho-Novum 10/11	ethinyl estradiol 35 mcg	norethindrone 0.5 mg (10 tablets)/ 1.0 mg (11 tablets)
Ovcon-50	ethinyl estradiol 50 mcg	norethindrone 1 mg
Ovcon-35	ethinyl estradiol 35 mcg	norethindrone 0.4 mg
Progestin dominant		
Loestrin 1.5/30	ethinyl estradiol 30 mcg	norethindrone 1.5 mg
Loestrin 1/20	ethinyl estradiol 20 mcg	norethindrone 1 mg
Lo/Ovral	ethinyl estradiol 30 mcg	norgestrel 0.3 mg
Norlestrin 2.5/50	ethinyl estradiol 50 mcg	norethindrone 2.5 mg
Ovral	ethinyl estradiol 50 mcg	norgestrel 0.5 mg
Progestin only		
Micronor	—	norethindrone 0.35 mg
Nor-Q.D.	—	norethindrone 0.35 mg
Ovrette	—	norgestrel 0.075 mg

cially true concerning the cardiovascular complications such as stroke, thromboembolic disease, heart attack, and pulmonary embolism. Other side effects of these agents include bleeding irregularities, nausea, vomiting, changes in libido, optic neuritis, depletion of vitamin B_6, chloasma, increased incidence of gallbladder disease, decreased glucose tolerance, and permanent infertility.

Contraindications and Cautions. Birth control tablets should not be taken during pregnancy or while breast feeding. They should not be used by individuals with active neoplastic disease or a history of neoplastic disease involving the breast or the genital organs. They should not be used (or be used with close monitoring) if the individual has a history of cardiovascular disease, migraine headaches, or diabetes.

NURSING IMPLICATIONS

- If patient forgets a dose, she should take it as soon as remembered, unless it is near the time for the next dose. In this instance, take it on time and without doubling the amount. If 2 days are missed, other means of birth control should be used until the next cycle starts.
- Teach monthly self-examination of breast; same day each month after menses.
- Instruct patients to report the following symptoms of thromboembolic disorders immediately: tenderness, swelling, redness in extremities, sudden severe headache or chest pain, change in vision, shortness of breath. Report to physician immediately.
- Pyridoxine (vitamin B_6) levels are lowered by estrogens. Supplements may be taken.
- Birth control tablets must be discontinued during pregnancy; they cause birth defects.
- Yearly gynecologic check-ups (pap smears) are advised.

OTHER AGENTS

Two other agents that are used in women are clomiphene (Clomid) and danazol (Danocrine). Clomiphene is a nonsteroidal drug with antiestrogenic properties and is used to induce ovulation in nonovulatory women. Its action involves stimulating an increased production of the gonadotropins, which leads to the maturation of many follicles in the ovaries and ovulation. Individuals who are given this agent usually will have multiple births, ovarian enlargements, hot flashes, nausea, abnormal uterine bleeding, and breast enlargement.

Danazol is a synthetic agent with no estrogenic or progestinic activity; it does have, however, mild androgenic effects. It suppresses the release of the gonadotropins; this disrupts the normal menstrual cycle resulting in nonovulation and amenorrhea. This action stops the pain and progression of endometriosis. This agent does have a virilizing effect. Changes such as deepening of the voice, oily skin, acne, clitoral enlargement, and hirsutism are observed and can be very disturbing to the individual. In addition, the cost for the treatment regimen is very expensive.

Androgens and Anabolic Steroids

The principal androgenic hormone in the male is testosterone, which is synthesized in and secreted by the Leydig cells of the testes. The principal effect of the androgenic hormones is in the development of secondary male characteristics. In addition, they possess an anabolic function that promotes growth and muscular development. Agents have been synthesized that predominantly have this anabolic activity, the so-called anabolics or anabolic steroids. The use of these agents among athletes and body builders has been the source of much concern about the health of the individual and the fairness of their use in competitive sports.

Action and Fate. These hormones, both the androgens and the anabolic hormones, act in a fashion similar to the steroids and the female hormones. They must penetrate the cells of the target tissues and there complex with their specific receptors, enter the nucleus, and there direct the synthesis of specific mRNAs. Both the androgenic and anabolic effect of these hormones cause the development and maintenance of the male secondary sex characteristics. The androgenic effect is primarily responsible for the growth spurt in adolescents and for growth termination. They increase erythropoiesis and they promote vascularization and darkening of the skin while the anabolic activity increases the production of protein and muscle tissue mass.

These agents are metabolized in the liver and excreted in the urine.

Uses. Androgens are used as replacement therapy in males who are deficient, i.e., male climacteric and postpubertal cryptorchism. In women, androgens may be used to treat postpartum breast pain and enlargement and in certain inoperable breast cancers. The agents with primarily anabolic effects are used to reverse the degenerative effects of prolonged debilitating states such as severe burns, paraplegia, and extensive surgery, and certain refractory anemias. They may also be used to retard osteoporosis. They are not indicated for increasing body mass.

Side and Adverse Effects. Both agents, the anabolics and the androgens, have very similar side effects. The following effects are seen in both sexes with both agents: they can cause increased libido, skin flushing, vascularization, and acne. They can cause sodium and water retention and GI upset. In females there is

TABLE 12–3. EXAMPLES OF SOME ANDROGENIC AND ANABOLIC AGENTS

Generic Name	Trade Name	Route of Administration
Agents with both androgenic and anabolic effects		
fluoxymesterone	Halotestin	PO
methyltestosterone	Metandren	PO, buccal
	Oreton	
testosterone cypionate	Depo-Testosterone	IM (long-acting preparation)
testosterone enanthate	Delatestryl	IM (long-acting preparation)
testosterone propionate	—	IM (long-acting preparation)
Agents with primarily anabolic effects		
ethylestrenol	Maxibolin	PO
methandriol	Anabol	IM
oxandrolone	Anavar	PO
stanozolol	Dianabol	PO
	Winstrol	

suppression of ovulation, lactation, menstruation, and virilization, i.e., deepening of the voice, hirsutism, and clitoral enlargement. In postpubital males, they cause testicular atrophy, impotence, penal enlargement, premature epiphyseal closure, and also suppress sperm formation. Some agents can also cause liver damage. For those agents with primarily anabolic effects, their long-term use can lead to behavioral changes such as extreme aggressiveness and combativeness.

Contraindications and Cautions. These agents should not be used in women who are pregnant or breast feeding. They should not be used in males who have breast cancer. They should be used with great caution in individuals of either sex who have a history of cardiovascular, hepatic, or renal disease. They should be used cautiously in prepubertal males.

NURSING IMPLICATIONS

- Sodium and water retention occurs with drug therapy. This can cause peripheral and central edema and weight gain. Also can cause hypertension.
- Cardiac and liver function tests should be performed during therapy; serum cholesterol and calcium levels should be checked regularly as well.
- Drug therapy may enhance hypoglycemia. Instruct diabetic patients to report sweating, tremor, anxiety, and vertigo.
- Testosterone alters glucose tolerance test.
- Female patients may experience masculinization, i.e., hirsutism, deepening of voice, increased muscle mass. May cause acne.
- Male patients may experience gynecomastia, lactating breast, sterility, impotence, and painful erection. Behavioral changes can occur such as aggressiveness.
- Prepubertal or adolescent males should be monitored closely to avoid precocious sexual development and premature epiphyseal closure.

Review Questions

1. Oral contraceptives are contraindicated in women with:
   a. renal disease
   b. rheumatoid arthritis
   c. a history of stroke
   d. diabetes

2. DES (diethylstilbestrol), as a "morning-after" pill must be administered within _____ hours after intercourse.

3. There are two structural forms of estrogens—the steroidal type and the nonsteroidal type. Which one of the following estrogen preparations is of the nonsteroidal type?
   a. DES
   b. estradiol
   c. ethinyl estradiol
   d. mestranol

4. Estrogen-dependent breast tumors are treated with which one of the following:
   a. Provera
   b. Clomid
   c. Nolvadex
   d. DES

5. Which one of the following vitamins is recommended for a woman to take if she is on birth control tablets?
   a. B_1
   b. B_2
   c. B_6
   d. B_{12}

6. The effectiveness of birth control tablets in preventing pregnancy is not only because ovulation is inhibited but also because there is(are):
   a. a decrease in sex drive
   b. changes in the cervical mucosa
   c. an increase in sex drive
   d. none of the above

7. The nausea that is sometimes experienced when taking birth control tablets is caused by the _____ component.
   a. estrogen
   b. progesterone

8. Which one of the following can be used to treat primary amenorrhea (i.e., interruption of the normal menstrual cycle because the individual did not ovulate)?
   a. Provera
   b. DES
   c. norethindrone
   d. norgestrel

9. Mood changes can occur in those individuals taking birth control tablets. These changes in mood are probably due to a decreased level in the body of which one of the following vitamins?
   a. B_1
   b. B_2
   c. B_6
   d. B_{12}

10–13. Matching:

Drug	Effect
10. ____ Dianabol	a. stimulates ovulation
11. ____ Provera	b. postmenopausal estrogen supplement
12. ____ Clomiphen	c. used for primary amenorrhea
13. ____ Premarin	d. anabolic steroid

14. Anabolic steroids can be used:
   a. to increase muscle mass

    b. to treat certain anemias
    c. to treat osteoporosis
    d. all of the above

15. Androgenic hormones are available as:
    a. buccal tablets
    b. pellets that can be implanted SQ
    c. parenterals for IM injections suspended in oil
    d. all of the above

=13=

Hypoglycemic Agents

Diabetes mellitus is a metabolic disease characterized by higher than normal fasting blood glucose values. Diabetics can be one of two types: Type I, insulin dependent (IDDM) or Type II, noninsulin dependent (NIDDM). Individuals diagnosed as Type I produce no insulin, experience a fast onset of the disease (usually weeks) at an early age (under 30), and are prone to ketoacidosis. They are treated by administering insulin. Type II diabetics, on the other hand, have functioning pancreatic beta cells that do produce insulin, but they are not as responsive to increased levels of glucose as the normally functioning beta cells. The Type II individuals are usually obese and over 40. The onset of Type II diabetes mellitus is slow (months to years). Treatment of Type IIs may consist of diet alone or diet in combination with an oral hypoglycemic agent. If these approaches are insufficient in controlling the glucose level, insulin can be added to the regimen. In no case, however, will an oral hypoglycemic agent be used in a Type I diabetic.

In both types of diabetics, pathological changes occur in the capillary basement membrane. A thickening occurs and it is this change that is thought to be responsible for many of the long-term complications associated with diabetes, i.e., premature atherosclerosis, glomerulosclerosis, retinopathy, neuropathy, and ulceration and gangrene of the extremities.

Treatment of each type of diabetes mellitus will be discussed separately.

TYPE I DIABETES MELLITUS

Type I diabetics are treated by administering insulin. Insulin is a hormone produced and secreted by the beta cells located in the islets of Langerhans in the pancreas. It is composed of two amino acid chains linked to each other by sulfur bonds. Commercial preparations are prepared by isolating insulin from the pancreas of beef and pork, with pork insulin bearing a closer resemblance to the amino acid sequence of human insulin.* Recent technological advances have produced (1) more highly purified (single source, single peak preparations); (2) allowed amino acid substitution in pork insulin making it identical to human insulin in amino acid sequence (semisynthetic preparations); and (3) a synthetic human insulin produced by bacteria modified by genetic engineering (recombinant DNA insulin).

The basic pharmacological action of all insulins, regardless of the source, is similar. The differences involved the onset, peak, and duration of action of the various preparations. These variations exist among the three different types of insulin because of varying particle size of the insulin complex. The larger the complex, the slower the onset and the longer the duration action. These differ-

---

* For those interested in a detailed account of the discovery of insulin, the book *The Discovery of Insulin* by Michael Bliss, published by University of Chicago Press, is an excellent account of this very important event.

ences are accomplished by complexing the insulin with a protein (protamine) in the presence of zinc in a buffered solution (NPH, PZI) or precipitating the insulin with zinc in another type of buffered solution (semilente, lente, and ultralente preparations). With all the advances made in insulin production, there are numerous insulin preparations available. These are listed in Table 13–1.

Action and Fate. When injected parenterally, insulin will produce the metabolic effects produced normally by the pancreatic beta cells. Insulin is needed for carbohydrate transport into various tissues in the body where it is used as a

TABLE 13–1. INSULIN PREPARATIONS

Preparation	Trade Name	Manufacturer	Source	Concentration (units/ml)
Rapid-acting preparations				
Insulin injection (regular insulin, crystalline zinc insulin)	Regular Iletin I	Lilly	Beef/pork	U40 and U100[b]
	Insulin Injection		Pork	U40 and U100
	Regular Iletin II	Lilly	Pure pork or pure beef	U100
	Velosulin[a]	Nordisk	Pork	U100
	Mixtard[a]	Nordisk	Pork	U100
	Regular Purified Pork[a]	Squibb/Novo	Pork	U100
Prompt insulin zinc suspension (semilente)	Semilente Iletin	Lilly	Beef/pork	U40 and U100
	Semilente Insulin	Squibb/Novo	Beef	U40 and U100
	Semilente Purified Pork[a]	Squibb/Novo	Pork	U100
Regular human insulin injection	Humalin R	Lilly	Recombinant DNA	U100
Regular semisynthetic human insulin injection	Novolin R	Squibb/Novo	Pork (with amino acid substitution)	U100
Intermediate-acting preparations				
Isophane insulin injection (NPH)	NPH Iletin	Lilly	Beef/pork	U40 and U100
	Novolin N	Squibb/Novo	Pork	U40 and U100
	NPH Iletin II[a]	Lilly	Pure pork or pure beef	U100
	NPH Purified Pork[a]	Squibb/Novo	Pork	U100
	Insulatard[a]	Nordisk	Pork	U100
	Purified NPH[a]		Beef	U100
Insulin zinc suspension (lente)	Lente Iletin I	Lilly	Beef/pork	U40 and U100
	Lente Insulin		Beef	U40 and U100
	Lente Iletin II[a]	Lilly	Pure pork or pure beef	U100
	Lente Purified Pork[a]	Squibb/Novo	Pork	U100
	Lentard[a]	Squibb/Novo	Beef/pork	U100
	Purified Lente[a]	Squibb/Novo	Beef	U100
NPH isophane human insulin suspension	Humalin N	Lilly	Recombinant DNA	U100
Lente semisynthetic human insulin suspension	Novolin L	Squibb/Novo	Pork (with amino acid substitution)	U100
Lente human insulin suspension	Humalin L	Lilly	Recombinant DNA	U100
Long-acting preparations				
Protamine zinc insulin suspension (PZI)	Protamine Zinc Iletin I	Lilly	Beef/pork	U40 and U100
	Protamine Zinc Insulin	Squibb/Novo	Beef/pork	U40 and U100
	Protamine Zinc Iletin II[a]	Lilly	Pure pork or pure beef	U100
Extended zinc insulin suspension (ultralente)	Ultralente Iletin I	Lilly	Beef/pork	U40 and U100
	Ultralente Insulin	Squibb/Novo	Beef	U100
	Ultralente Purified Beef[a]	Squibb/Novo	Beef	U100
Ultralente human insulin suspension	Humalin U	Lilly	Recombinant DNA	U100

[a] Purified preparations.
[b] An insulin with a concentration of 40 units/ml is referred to as U40 insulin. An insulin with a concentration of 100 units/ml is referred to as U100 insulin.

source of energy (Fig. 13–1). Insulin is not needed, however, for glucose transport into neural tissue, erthrocytes, and kidney cells. It is also not needed for glucose transport into the liver, but it is needed for its conversion to glycogen for storage. Insulin also affects fat and protein metabolism. It stimulates the formation of fatty tissue (lipogenesis) and prevents fatty tissue breakdown (lipolysis) and the release of free fatty acids. Insulin also promotes the transport of amino acids into various tissues and their conversion into protein. Figure 13–2 shows the metabolic alterations that occur when insulin is not present. In addition to its metabolic role, insulin has also been found to promote the intracellular migration of potassium and magnesium ions.

Insulin has a short plasma half-life in the body, about 3 to 5 minutes. It is primarily metabolized in the liver with less than 2 percent excreted in the urine unchanged.

Uses. Insulin is used to normalize blood glucose levels in individuals who are classed as Type I diabetics and in those Type II diabetics who are not responsive to hypoglycemic agents or diet. Regular insulin may be added to hyperalimentation solutions to insure proper use of the glucose and it may also be used to promote the intracellular shift of potassium ions in hyperkalemia. Regular insulin is the only preparation that can be administered intravenously, therefore it is the one used in hyperalimentation solutions or in reversing diabetic ketoacidosis.

Side and Adverse Effects. Side and adverse effects of insulin preparations involve hypersensitivity reactions at injection site, or generalized hypoglycemia, and hypertrophy or atrophy at an injection site that is used repeatedly.

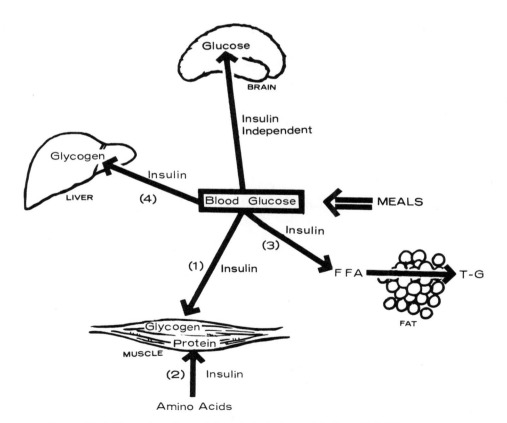

Figure 13–1. Normal postprandial carbohydrate metabolism. High blood glucose leads to the release of insulin, which in turn leads to uptake of glucose and amino acids by peripheral tissues. (*From Herfindal, ET [ed]: Clinical Pharmacy and Therapeutics. Baltimore, Md, The Williams and Wilkins Company, 1975, with permission.*)

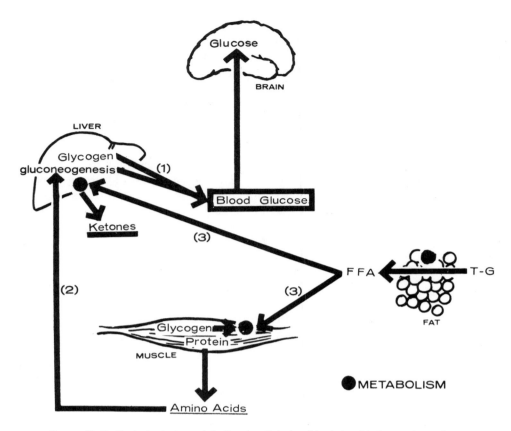

Figure 13-2. Carbohydrate metabolism for diabetes. Meals lead to hyperglycemia; a deficiency of insulin leads to increased systemic glucose production and decreased uptake of glucose by peripheral tissues. (*From Herfindal, ET [ed]: Clinical Pharmacy and Therapeutics, Baltimore, Md, The Williams and Wilkins Company, copyright 1975, with permission.*)

Contraindications and Cautions. Hypersensitivity to foreign animal proteins found in insulin preparations.

TYPE II DIABETES MELLITUS

Type II diabetics differ from Type I diabetics in that they have retained the ability to synthesize insulin, but the amount secreted is much less than what is needed to use the glucose present and the response of the beta cells may be somewhat delayed. For this reason, Type II diabetics can be treated by reducing their carbohydrate intake. If this is not sufficient, an oral hypoglycemic agent is given.

Action and Fate. The oral hypoglycemic agents are classified chemically as sulfonylureas. They are related to the sulfonamides but do not possess antibacterial activity. These agents lower blood glucose levels by stimulating pancreatic beta cells to synthesize and release insulin. The second generation agents, it is thought, also increase insulin receptor sensitivity to the hormone.

These agents may either be excreted unchanged by the kidneys or metabolized to either active or inactive metabolites in the liver, which are excreted. For individual agents see Table 13-2.

Uses. No therapeutic action is seen with these agents if there are no functional beta cells present in the pancreas. Therefore the oral hypoglycemic agents are used in the management of Type II, noninsulin-development diabetics in con-

TABLE 13–2. ORAL HYPOGLYCEMIC AGENTS

Generic Name	Trade Name(s)	Dosage range (mg/24 hr)	Half-life ($t_{1/2}$) (hr)	Duration of Action (hr)	Metabolism
First generation agents					
tolbutamide	Orinase	500–3000[a]	4–7	6–12	Metabolized in liver to less active metabolite, excreted via urine
chlorpropamide	Diabinese	100–500[b]	35	24–72	Up to 60% excreted unchanged via kidneys
acetohexamide	Dymelor	250–1500[c]	3.5–8	12–18+	Metabolized in liver, metabolite more active, excreted via kidneys
tolazamide	Tolinase	100–1000[c]	7	12–16+	Metabolized in liver to less active metabolite, excreted via kidneys
Second generation agents					
glyburide	DiaBeta Micronaise	2.5–20[c]	7–10	10–24	Metabolized in liver to less active metabolite, excreted via kidneys and bile
glipizide	Glucotrol	2.5–40[c]	3–7	6–24	Metabolized in liver to inactive metabolite, excreted via kidneys

[a] Given in daily divided doses.
[b] Given in a single daily dose.
[c] Given in either a single daily dose or in divided daily doses.

junction with dietary control and weight reduction. They also may be used with insulin in certain Type II individuals in order to stabilize them.

Side and Adverse Effects. The sulfonylureas can cause a number of dermatologic reactions including pruritis, erythema, urticaria, and photosensitivity. Their use is also associated with gastrointernal upsets (nausea, anorexia, heartburn, and constipation or diarrhea). Other adverse effects include various hemotologic disorders, antabuse effect with alcohol, and hypoglycemia.

Contraindications and Cautions. Individuals with known hypersensitivity to sulfonamides and Type I diabetics should avoid sulfonylureas. Cautious use in those with renal or liver function impairment. Safe use during pregnancy not established.

NURSING IMPLICATIONS

General

- Time, content, and number of meals as suggested by dietitian must be adhered to.
- Repeated episodes of hypoglycemia will cause permanent brain damage. Teach individual to recognize signs and symptoms of hypoglycemia (Table 13–3).
- Repeated episodes of hyperglycemia may hasten the onset of long-term complications. Stress importance of taking medication as directed and monitoring blood glucose levels (Table 13–5).
- Both types of diabetics should be taught proper personal hygiene; skin, foot, and dental care; and infection prevention.
- Know medications that alter carbohydrate metabolism and those that antagonize insulin (Table 13–4).
- Increase or decrease in exercise regimen will alter medication requirements.

TABLE 13–3. SIGNS AND SYMPTOMS OF DIABETIC COMA (HYPERGLYCEMIA) AND INSULIN REACTION (HYPOGLYCEMIA)

Early Signs	Later Signs
Diabetic coma (hyperglycemia)	
Polyuria	Kussmaul breathing
Polydipsia	Signs of dehydration
Headache	Fruity odor of breath
Nausea	Cherry-colored lips
Sugar in the urine	Elevated blood glucose levels
Fatigue	Positive C and A
Mental dullness	Incoherent
	Coma
Insulin reaction (hypoglycemia)	
Headache	Blurred vision
Sudden hunger	Dilated pupils
Diphoresis	Poor coordination
Inappropriate behavior	Abdominal pain
Slight confusion	Nausea
Shakiness	Sugar-free urine
Restlessness	Decreased blood glucose levels
	Convulsions
	Coma

Insulin

- Regular insulin is the only type that can be given IV or added to an IV infusion.
- Insulin may be purchased without a prescription; a prescription may be needed for the syringe and needle, however.
- Insulin in use is stable at room temperature up to 1 month; refrigerate stock supply.
- Avoid injecting cold insulin; can lead to lipodystrophy and poor absorption.

  Before administration: Examine vial before use; do not use if solution is discolored.
  Check expiration date on label; discard out-of-date preparations.
  Insulins should not be mixed unless specified by a physician.
  Always use coordinating syringe with strength of insulin being used.
  Rotate insulin suspensions gently to disperse particles. DO NOT SHAKE WELL.

- Insulin is generally administered 15 to 30 minutes before a meal; it is very important to administer insulin about the same time daily.

TABLE 13–4. INSULIN–DRUG INTERACTIONS

Drug	Effect
alcohol anabolic steroids monoamine oxidase inhibitors guanethidine salicylates (large doses)	Enhance hypoglycemic effect of insulin
dextrothyroxine corticosteroids epinephrine oral contraceptives estrogen preparations phenothiazines	Antagonize insulin effect
propanolol (Inderal)	Interferes with carbohydrate metabolism and masks symptoms of hypoglycemia
thiazide diuretics furosemide (Lasix) ethacrynic acid (Edecrin)	Elevate fasting blood sugar levels

- Rotate injection sites to prevent atrophy of tissue. If patient is engaged in active sports, it has been suggested that injection be rotated in the abdomen rather than into a muscle.
- Monitor patient for signs and symptoms of anaphalactic reaction to new types of insulin: closure of throat, decreased blood pressure, increased heart rate, skin cool and clammy.
- Blood testing is replacing urine testing as a more accurate reflection of endogenous glucose level.

Oral Agents

- Because of the danger of nocturnal hypoglycemia, especially with long-acting agents, oral agents should not be taken at bedtime unless so specified.
- Oral agents may cause photosensitivity in some individuals. Advise individual to avoid direct sunlight or to use a sunscreen.
- Teach patients the importance of recognizing signs and symptoms of an allergic reaction: rash, pruritis.
- Agents often cause gastrointestinal upsets; they should be taken with meals.

Review Questions

1. Insulin is used in the body to:
   a. promote fatty acid catabolism
   b. inhibit the conversion of glucose to glycogen
   c. stimulate gluconeogenesis
   d. facilitate glucose transport across membranes

2. Sites of injection for insulin are rotated in order to:
   a. decrease allergic reactions
   b. obtain blood levels
   c. prevent lipodystrophy
   d. constrict blood vessels

3. Hypoglycemia can occur if the normal dose of insulin is given and a meal is missed. Symptoms of hypoglycemia include:
   a. leg cramps/blurred vision
   b. polyuria/polydipsia
   c. headache/tremors
   d. tinnitus/diaphoresis

4. If an insulin-dependent diabetic is given prednisone 50 mg twice a day (a corticosteroid), his or her normal dose would probably need to be:
   a. decreased
   b. increased

5. An insulin-dependent diabetic develops a urinary tract infection. The regular dose of insulin would be:
   a. decreased
   b. increased

6. Mrs. Smith, an insulin-dependent diabetic, has started a fitness program which includes jogging. Her regular dose of insulin will probably need to be:
   a. decreased
   b. increased

7. Which one of the following drugs can mask symptoms of hypoglycemia in addition to causing hypoglycemia?
   a. estrogens
   b. propranolol

    c. furosemide
    d. hydrochlorothiazide

8. The oral hypoglycemic drug, tolbutamide, would *not* be used if which one of the following conditions were present?
    a. cirrhosis
    b. cardiovascular disease
    c. cataracts
    d. oliguria

9. Which one of the following oral hypoglycemic agents is about 60 percent excreted unchanged by the kidneys?
    a. acetohexamide
    b. tolazamide
    c. chlorpropamide
    d. tolbutamide

10. Which one of the following has the longest half-life ($t_{1/2}$) and should be dosed once a day?
    a. acetohexamide
    b. tolazamide
    c. chlorpropamide
    d. tolbutamide

11. Side effects associated with oral hypoglycemic drugs include:
    a. rashes
    b. gastrointestinal upsets
    c. hypoglycemia
    d. all of the above

12–16. Matching:

Insulin

12. _____ Regular
13. _____ PZI
14. _____ Semilente
15. _____ NPH
16. _____ Lente

Type of Action

a. short acting
b. intermediate acting
c. long acting

17–20. Matching:

Generic Name

17. _____ chlorpropamide
18. _____ tolbutamide
19. _____ glyburide
20. _____ glipizide

Trade Name

a. Glucotrol
b. Diabinese
c. Orinase
d. Micronase, DiaBeta

=14=

Agents for Peptic Ulcers

Peptic ulcer disease occurs in about 10 to 15 percent of the population. Both gastric and duodenal ulcers are labeled as peptic ulcers even though their respective etiologies are different. Individuals with gastric ulcers are thought to have gastric stasis and poor emptying of contents. This leads to irritation of the gastric mucosa, which in turn lowers the resistance of the mucosa to the corrosive effects of even minimal amounts of hydrochloric acid and pepsin. Individuals with duodenal ulcers usually have higher than average production of hydrochloric acid. Certain medications can also be the cause of peptic ulcer formation (Table 14–1).

Management of peptic ulcer disease consists of changes in diet and lifestyle. In addition, individuals are given one or more of the agents that either inhibit the secretion of hydrochloric acid, neutralize or increase gastric pH, or produce a protective substance that protects the ulcer from hydrochloric acid and pepsin. See Table 14–2 for a list of agents used in the treatment of peptic ulcers.

H$_2$-RECEPTOR ANTAGONISTS

Action and Fate. These agents are competitive inhibitors of the H$_2$ receptors located on the parietal cells. This action inhibits the gastrin- and histamine-induced acid secretion in the stomach. This action not only reduces the concentration, but also the volume of the acid produced.

Cimetidine is metabolized in the liver prior to being excreted in the urine; ranitidine is excreted primarily unchanged.

Uses. Both agents are used to treat duodenal ulcer disease and pathological gastrointestinal hypersecretion disease. In addition, cimetidine is also indicated in the prevention of duodenal ulcer recurrence.

Side and Adverse Effects. Headache, tiredness, diarrhea, constipation, dizziness, rash, muscle pain, gynecomastia, and impotence have been reported for both agents but less frequently for ranitidine.

Contraindications and Cautions. These agents should be used with caution in the elderly and in individuals with kidney and liver impairment. Safe use of both agents during pregnancy, in women with child-bearing potential, and nursing women not established.

NURSING IMPLICATIONS

• Monitor the elderly for mental confusion and dizziness.
• Gynecomastia may occur after 1 month therapy with cimetidine.

135

TABLE 14–1. DRUGS THAT ARE ASSOCIATED WITH THE FORMATION OF PEPTIC ULCERS

Generic Name	Trade Name
alcohol	—
aspirin	—
indomethacin	Indocin
methotrexate	Mexate
phenylbutazone	Butazolidin
reserpine	Serpasil
steroids	Various preparations

- Both agents may be given with food.
- Avoid enteric-coated medications during treatment with these agents. Increasing gastric pH will prematurely dissolve the protective coating exposing the gastric mucosa to irritating medication. Examples of enteric-coated tablets are bisacodyl, methenamine, and enteric-coated aspirin.

ANTACIDS

Action, Fate, and Uses. Antacids are used in the treatment of peptic ulcer disease to neutralize or increase the pH of the stomach. This action inhibits the corrosive effect of pepsin thus relieving pain and promoting the healing of the ulcer. Clinically useful antacids contain aluminum, calcium, and magnesium either as hydroxides or other salt forms (Table 14–3).

Most antacids are not systemically absorbed except dihydroxyaluminum, sodium carbonate, and to a small extent, magnesium hydroxide.

Side and Adverse Effects. Antacids that are systemically absorbed can produce systemic alkalosis. The principal adverse effect of aluminum-containing products is diarrhea, and for magnesium-containing products, constipation.

TABLE 14–2. AGENTS USED IN THE TREATMENT OF PEPTIC ULCERS

Generic Name	Trade Name	Comments
Antacids		
Aluminum-containing products		
aluminum carbonate gel, basic	Basaljel	Not systemically absorbed
aluminum hydroxide	ALternaGEL	Not systemically absorbed
	Alu-Cap	
	Alu-Tab	
	Amphojel	
	Dialume	
aluminum phosphate	Phosphaljel	Not systemically absorbed
dihydroxyaluminum sodium	Rolaids	Some systemic absorption
Calcium-containing products		
calcium carbonate	Alka-2	Not systemically absorbed, associated with mild alkalosis
	Titralac	
	Tums	
Magnesium-containing products		
magnesium hydroxide	Milk of Magnesia	Some systemic absorption, also used as a laxative
H₂-receptor blockers		
cimetidine	Tagamet	PO and IV dose the same
ranitidine	Zantac	Dosed twice a day for PO administration, IV dose is less than PO dose
famotidine	Pepcid	Dosed once a day PO, or twice a day PO or IV
Miscellaneous agents		
sucralfate	Carafate	Local healing action

TABLE 14–3. FORMULATIONS OF SOME ANTACID MIXTURES

Product Name	Formulation
Aludrox, Maalox	Aluminum hydroxide/magnesium hydroxide
Camalox	Aluminum hydroxide/magnesium hydroxide, calcium carbonate
Mylanta	Aluminum hydroxide/magnesium hydroxide/simethicone
Riopan	Magaldrate

Contraindications and Cautions. Use of those antacids that contain aluminum should be restricted in individuals with a history of sensitivity to aluminum, low serum phosphate, and decreased bowel motility. Calcium-containing antacids are not used in those with an elevated serum calcium level, renal calculi, and decreased bowel motility. Indications that limit the use of magnesium-containing products are abdominal pain, nausea, vomiting, and diarrhea. Cautious use is recommended for all products in individuals on sodium-restricted diets unless the product is designed specifically for use with a low-sodium-content diet.

NURSING IMPLICATIONS

- Liquid products are more efficient in neutralizing stomach pH than tablets.
- Aluminum and magnesium products may be alternated to balance the constipation or diarrhea caused by each agent.
- Be sure to advise patient to shake suspensions well.
- Antacid dose should be followed by water to ensure passage into stomach.
- Do not administer antacids with enteric-coated tablets. Increasing the pH of the stomach will prematurely dissolve the protective coating causing gastric irritation by the medication. Examples of medications that are enteric coated are bisacodyl, methenamine, and enteric-coated aspirin.
- Use low-sodium preparations for patients on salt-restricted intake.

MISCELLANEOUS AGENT: SUCRALFATE

Action, Fate, and Uses. Sucralfate acts in a way totally unlike the other antiulcer agents. Once the medication is in the stomach, it reacts with hydrochloride acid to form a viscous, paste-like substance that adheres to the gastrointestinal mucosa forming a protective barrier. This barrier prevents further mucosal corrosion by hydrochloric acid, pepsin, and bile acid.

It is not absorbed systemically and causes minimal side effects. Sucralfate is indicated in the treatment of duodenal ulcers. Safe use during pregnancy has not been established.

NURSING IMPLICATIONS

- Give sucralfate 1 hour before meals.
- A suspension can be prepared by the pharmacist for nasogastric tube administration. Do not attempt to crush tablet.
- Sucralfate decreases the absorption of cimetidine, phenytoin, and tetracyclines.

Review Questions

1. Which one of the following agents reacts with hydrochloric acid to form a viscous locally protective barrier in the stomach?
   a. Basaljel
   b. Phosphajel

   c. Tagamet
   d. Carafate

2. You should advise the patient to follow each dose of an antacid with:
   a. milk
   b. dilute solution of sodium bicarbonate
   c. water
   d. carbonated beverage

3. The outer layer of enteric-coated tablets will prematurely dissolve if the pH of the stomach is above 7.
   a. True
   b. False

4–10. Match the statements given in Column A with the antacids listed in Column B. Answers may be used more than once.

Column A	Column B
4. ＿＿causes constipation	a. Milk of Magnesia
5. ＿＿causes diarrhea	b. ranitidine
6. ＿＿exerts local healing action	c. sucralfate
7. ＿＿PO and IV dose may be the same	d. cimetidine
8. ＿＿oral dosing frequency is BID	e. aluminum hydroxide
9. ＿＿may cause some systemic alkalosis	
10. ＿＿gynecomastia can occur	

List five drugs that are associated with the formation of peptic ulcers.

11. ＿＿＿＿＿＿＿＿＿

12. ＿＿＿＿＿＿＿＿＿

13. ＿＿＿＿＿＿＿＿＿

14. ＿＿＿＿＿＿＿＿＿

15. ＿＿＿＿＿＿＿＿＿

15

Antidiarrheal Agents and Laxatives

ANTIDIARRHEALS

Diarrhea is characterized by loose stools with excessive fluid and increased weight. Diarrhea is also associated with an increased number of daily bowel movements of at least three a day. There are a number of factors that can cause diarrhea; these include infection, food intolerance, alteration of the normal gut flora, malabsorption syndrome, inflammatory bowel disease, and bowel tumors. Both acute (severe) diarrhea and chronic (mild) diarrhea are cause for concern. Both can cause an electrolyte imbalance and dehydration especially in infants, the elderly, and debilitated patients. In an otherwise healthy individual, acute diarrhea is usually self-limiting and treatment is optional. In acute or chronic diarrhea, treatment is aimed toward temporary relief for the patient until the primary cause is determined. Agents used to symptomatically treat diarrhea can be divided into three groups: opiates and opioids, anticholinergic antispasmotic agents, and absorbents (Tables 15–1 and 15–2).

Opiates and Opioids

Action and Fate. The opiates and their derivatives are probably the most effective and prompt-acting antidiarrheal agents. These agents act by inhibiting gastrointestinal peristaltic action, which in turn prolongs the transit time of the contents of the intestine. This in turn decreases the number of bowel movements per day and increases the consistency of the stools.

Uses. Opiates and opioids are used to treat acute, nonspecific diarrhea, and some cases of chronic diarrhea; and to reduce fecal volume in ileostomies.

Side and Adverse Effects. The more serious adverse effects of these agents, as discussed in Chapter 9, are not usually seen with the doses given for diarrhea. Usual complaints include constipation, dry mouth, drowsiness, dizziness, nausea, and vomiting.

Contraindications and Cautions. These agents should not be used in acute diarrhea caused by broad-spectrum antibiotics, poisons, or infectious organisms that penetrate the intestinal mucosal. It is important not to treat acute diarrhea in cases where a toxin is being secreted by the invading organism or a poison has been ingested until the toxic substance has been eliminated from the gastrointestinal tract. These agents should be used cautiously in hepatic impairment. The safe use of these agents during pregnancy, for nursing mothers, or for children has not been established.

TABLE 15-1. AGENTS USED TO SYMPTOMATICALLY TREAT DIARRHEA

Generic Name	Trade Name	Comments
Opiates and opioids		
diphenoxylate	In Lomotil with atropine	Do not exceed 8 tablets per day, CV controlled substance
loperamide	Imodium	Do not exceed 8 capsules per day
opium tincture (deodor-ized)	—	Dose range is 0.3–1 ml 4 times a day, not to exceed 6 ml per 24 hours, CII controlled substance
paregoric (camphorated opium tincture)	—	Dose range is 5–10 ml 4 times a day, CIII controlled substance
Other agents		
bismuth subsalicylate	Pepto-Bismol	May turn stool black, does not require a prescription

NURSING IMPLICATIONS

- Replacement of fluids and electrolytes may be necessary in severe cases of diarrhea based on electrolyte laboratory values.
- Instruct patient to avoid products that can worsen diarrhea such as dairy products, concentrated sweets, and cold drinks; and to maintain a bland diet until diarrhea subsides.
- All the opiates and one derivative are controlled substances. Tincture of opium is a CII; paregoric a CIII; and diphenoxylate a CV. Loperamide is not a controlled substance.

Anticholinergic Antispasmodic Agents

Action and Uses. These agents which are extracted from the Belladonna leaf are principally used to inhibit the spasms and hypermotility associated with diarrhea. The precautions, adverse reactions, and nursing implications are similar to other anticholinergic agents.

Absorbants

Action and Uses. Substances such as bismuth, kaolin, and pectin are classed as absorbants because of their ability to absorb toxins, bacteria, and viruses facilitating their excretion. In addition, bismuth is reported to provide a protective coating for the intestinal mucosa.

TABLE 15-2. COMBINATION PRODUCTS USED TO SYMPTOMATICALLY TREAT DIARRHEA

Product	Formulation
Donnagel	Kaolin Pectin Sodium benzoate Hyoscyamine Atropine
Donnagel PG	Same as above plus powdered opium (24 mg/30 ml)
Kaopectate	Kaolin Pectin
Infantol Pink	Bismuth subsalicylate Pectin Calcium carrageenan Zinc phenosulfonate Paregoric (0.078 ml/5 ml)
Parepectolin	Kaolin Pectin Paregoric (3.7 ml/30 ml)

Adverse Effects and Cautions. In general, these agents are safe but may interfere with the absorption of other therapeutic agents if given simultaneously. For this reason it is recommended that the absorbants be given 2 to 3 hours before or after the administration of the medication.

The use of absorbants is contraindicated in patients with obstruction lesions of the bowel and children under 3 years of age.

NURSING IMPLICATIONS

- Instruct the patients to carefully read the directions and not to exceed recommended doses.
- Bismuth preparations temporarily darken the tongue and stools.
- Some bismuth preparations contain salicylate, which may be contraindicated for some patients.
- Bismuth subsalicylate may be used prophylactically for travelers' diarrhea.

LAXATIVES

Laxatives are agents that promote bowel movements by various mechanisms. At one time laxatives were an integral part of the general treatment for many illnesses, and a good purge is still considered by some to be beneficial (Table 15–3). This coupled with the fact that laxatives are a nonlegend product that can be purchased freely by the consumer has led to their misuse and overuse. Chronic laxative use is not without serious effects. It can lead to electrolyte imbalance,

TABLE 15–3. COMMONLY USED LAXATIVES

Generic Name	Trade Name	Site of Action	Onset of Action (hr)
Bulk-forming agents			
calcium polycarbophil	Mitrolan	Small and large intestines	12–72
carboxymethylcellulose	In various products	Small and large intestines	12–72
methylcellulose	In various products	Small and large intestines	12–72
psyllium	Konsyl Metamucil	Small and large intestines	12–72
Osmotic agents			
glycerin suppository		Colon	0.25–1
magnesium citrate		Small and large intestines	0.5–3
magnesium hydroxide	Milk of Magnesia	Small and large intestines	0.5–3
magnesium sulfate		Small and large intestines	0.5–3
sodium biphosphate/ sodium phosphate	Fleet	As enema: colon	2–15 min
		Orally: small and large intestines	6–12
lactulose	Cephulac Chronulac	Colon	24–48
Stool softeners			
Surfactants			
docusate calcium	Surfak	Small and large intestines	12–72
docusate sodium	Colace	Small and large intestines	12–72
Lubricant			
mineral oil		Colon	6–8
Stimulants			
aloe	In various products	Colon	8–12
bisacodyl	Dulcolax Theralax	Colon	Suppository: 0.25–1 Tablet: 6–10
cascara sagrada		Colon	6–8
castor oil		Small intestine	2–6
danthron	Dorbane Modane	Colon	6–8
senna	Senokot	Colon	6–10
phenolphthalein	Ex-Lax Feen-a-Mint	Colon	6–8

fluid loss, depletion of oil-soluble vitamins, and dependence on these agents for regular bowel movements (the laxative habit).

Action and Fate. Laxatives are grouped according to their mechanisms of action. Each group will be discussed individually.

Bulk laxatives are considered to be the most physiologically normal agents. These agents stimulate intestinal activity and normalize stool consistency by retaining water in the lumen of the intestine. These products should be taken with a glass of water to prevent bowel obstruction. These agents are not absorbed systemically.

Osmotic laxatives are minimally absorbed systemically. They retain water in the lumen of the intestine by their osmotic action. This action adds fluid bulk to the stool facilitating excretion.

Stool softeners are of two types: lubricant (mineral oil) and surfactants (salts of dioctyl sulfosuccinate). Under normal conditions systemic absorption of mineral oil is minimal. It acts locally in the intestine to lubricate and soften the stools for easy evacuation. Surfactant-type laxatives soften stools by acting as emulsifying agents by promoting increased water retention in the intestine.

Stimulant or irritant laxatives actually increase the peristalic action of the intestines. These laxatives should be used only for specific indications. Their overuse will lead to dependence on these agents for regular bowel movements. These agents are systemically absorbed and they can be found in breast milk.

Uses. There are specific indications for the use of laxatives. These include the relief of constipation caused by opiates and opioids, medications with anticholinergic side effects, and atony of the bowel. Laxatives may be required by bedridden patients, postoperative patients, postmyocardial infarct patients in whom straining would not be desirable, and patients with hemorrhoids or fissures. They are also used to evacuate the gastrointestinal tract prior to radiographic procedures.

Side and Adverse Effects. Severe abdominal cramping and griping is associated with the stimulant type of laxative. Accumulation of bulk laxatives can occur if not taken with an adequate amount of water and may lead to esophageal, small intestine, gastric, or rectal obstruction. Magnesium salts can cause electrolyte imbalance and dehydration. Mineral oil can deplete the body of oil-soluble vitamins. Also, the repeated accidental aspiration of mineral oil can cause acute pneumonitis, chronic diffuse pneumonitis, or localized granulomas.

Contraindications and Cautions. Laxatives should not be used by individuals experiencing abdominal pain, nausea, and vomiting; fecal impaction; or intestinal obstruction or perforation. Products containing magnesium should not be used in patients with renal impairment. Bulk laxatives that are sugar free should be used for diabetics. Laxative use during pregnancy and while breast feeding should be under the direction of the physician.

NURSING IMPLICATIONS

- Instruct patients that prior to taking a laxative, it is important to consider the following: Is there adequate fluid intake? Are there proper dietary habits including adequate amounts of fresh fruits, vegetables, and fiber? Is there some type of daily exercise regimen?
- Laxatives should not be used during pregnancy or while breast feeding without medical supervision.
- Bisacodyl tablets should not be given with milk, antacids, or medications that elevate gastric pH. A basic pH in the stomach causes premature dissolution of the enteric coating causing gastric irritation.

- Avoid administering a stool softener with mineral oil. This combination promotes systemic absorption of the mineral oil.
- Phenolphthalein discolors alkaline urine pink/red.
- Advise patients not to use laxatives if there is abdominal pain, nausea, and vomiting.
- Overuse and abuse of laxatives will lead to the laxative habit and individuals should be encouraged to make dietary changes, such as increased fiber and fruit intake, to manage problems related to constipation.

Review Questions

1. Which of the following agents used for diarrhea may temporarily blacken the tongue and stools?
   a. Kaopectate
   b. Donnagel
   c. Pepto-Bismol
   d. Parepectolin

2. The class of antidiarrheal agents with the fastest onset of action is:
   a. anticholinergic agents
   b. absorbants
   c. opiates
   d. subsalicylates

3. The recommended maximum daily dose for Lomotil is:
   a. one tablet tid
   b. one tablet qid
   c. two tablets tid
   d. two tablets qid

4. Which one of the following antidiarrheal agents is classed as a schedule II substance?
   a. opium tincture
   b. Paregoric
   c. Lomotil
   d. Imodium

Give four contraindications for the use of antidiarrheal agents.

5. _____

6. _____

7. _____

8. _____

9. _____ may be used to treat travelers' diarrhea.
   a. Donnagel PG
   b. Pepto-Bismol
   c. Kaopectate
   d. Parepectolin

10. Define laxative habit.

Give three changes in life style the individual can make in order to promote normal bowel function.

11. _____

12. _____

13. _____

14. Which one of the following classes of laxatives is the most physiologically normal?
    a. stimulants
    b. osmotic laxatives
    c. stool softeners
    d. bulk laxatives

15–19. Match the characteristics listed in Column A with the laxative type listed in Column B.

Column A

15. ____enteric-coated tablet
16. ____repeated aspiration causes pneumonitis
17. ____causes discoloration of alkaline urine
18. ____should not be simultaneously administered with mineral oil
19. ____repeated use causes oil-soluble vitamin depletion

Column B

a. mineral oil
b. phenolphthalein
c. stool softeners
d. bisacodyl

20. Patients with renal impairment should *not* use products containing:
    a. methylcellulose
    b. magnesium
    c. docusate
    d. danthron

21–30. Match the laxative name listed in Column A with the class that is most applicable listed in Column B.

Column A

21. ____Metamucil
22. ____Cephulac
23. ____Modane
24. ____Dulcolax
25. ____Castor Oil
26. ____Cascara Sagrada
27. ____Fleet
28. ____Colace
29. ____Surfak
30. ____Milk of Magnesia

Column B

a. bulk-forming agents
b. osmotic agents
c. stool softener (surfactant)
d. stool softener (lubricant)
e. stimulants

=16=

Anti-infective Agents

Penicillins

In 1928, it was observed that the growth of certain bacteria was inhibited in cultures contaminated with the mold *Penicillium notatum*. The benefit of this important observation was not fully realized, however, until the 1940s when penicillin, the inhibiting substance, could be produced in sufficient quantities at an affordable price for general use. Even though the prototype, penicillin G (pen G), was very effective and a lifesaving antibiotic, it did have some disadvantages. Pen G has a relatively narrow spectrum of activity; it is destroyed by the acid in the stomach (acid labile) making its absorption erratic; and with continued use, it has become ineffective against resistant strains of bacteria, particularly *Staphylococcus*. The resistance that has occurred is one in which the bacteria produce an enzyme, penicillinase, which is capable of destroying the antibiotic. These disadvantages led to the development of semisynthetic penicillin derivatives. These derivatives can be divided into two subgroups according to their major advantage over pen G, the penicillinase-resistant derivatives, and the broad-spectrum derivatives (Table 16–1). Also included in Table 16–1 are repository preparations of pen G. These preparations are combined with either benzathine or procaine and are specifically formulated to slowly release pen G from the intramuscular injection site. This type of formulation will maintain therapeutic blood levels for a prolonged period of time after one injection. The penicillins are an important group of antibiotics. They are extremely useful and are still the drug of choice for certain infections.

Action and Fate. All the penicillins share a common mechanism of action. They inhibit the synthesis of precursor molecules essential in the synthesis of the cell wall of certain bacteria. These agents are most effective against rapidly growing and dividing bacteria. At therapeutic blood levels, the penicillins are considered to be bactericidal; at lower blood levels they are bacteriostatic.

Penicillins do not undergo metabolic transformation and therefore are excreted unchanged by renal tubular secretion via the urine. Excretion of these agents can be delayed in individuals with immature or impaired renal function. Penicillins cross the placenta and will appear in breast milk.

Uses. The uses of penicillin vary according to the group. Pen G and penicillin V are primarily effective against gram-positive cocci, gram-negative cocci, gram-positive and gram-negative bacilli, spirochetes, and actinomycetes. Pen G is the drug of choice for gonorrhea and is still effective in treating primary, secondary, or latent syphilis that is less than 1 year in duration. The penicillinase-resistant derivatives are effective against gram-positive cocci and several strains of *Staphylococcus*. The broad-spectrum derivatives have an extended spectrum of activity

145

TABLE 16–1. PENICILLINS

Generic Name	Trade Name(s)	Stability in Acid	Spectrum of Activity	Penicillinase Resistant	Route of Administration
Natural and semisynthetic derivatives					
penicillin G (benzyl penicillin)	Pentids	Poor	Narrow	No	PO, IV, IM
penicillin VK (phenoxymethyl penicillin)	Pen-Vee K V-Cillin K	Good	Narrow	No No	PO
Penicillinase-resistant penicillins					
cloxacillin	Tegopen	Good	Narrow	Yes	PO, IV, IM
dicloxacillin	Dynapen	Good	Narrow	Yes	PO
methicillin	Staphcillin	Poor	Narrow	Yes	IV, IM
nafcillin	Unipen	Good	Narrow	Yes	PO
oxacillin	Bactocill Prostaphlin	Good	Narrow	Yes	PO, IV, IM
Broad-spectrum penicillin derivatives					
amoxicillin	Amoxil Larotid Polymox	Excellent	Broad	No	PO
ampicillin	Omnipen Polycillin Principen	Fair	Broad	No	PO, IV, IM
carbenicillin					
disodium	Geopen Pyopen	Poor	Broad	No	IV, IM
indanyl sodium	Geocillin	Good	Broad	No	PO
ticarcillin	Ticar	Poor	Broad	No	IV, IM
piperacillin	Pipracil	Poor	Broad	No	IV, IM
Repository preparations					
benzathine penicillin G	Crysticillin A.S.	Poor	Narrow	No	IM
procaine penicillin G	Bicillin	Poor	Narrow	No	IM

that includes gram-negative rods. In addition, ampicillin and amoxicillin are effective against *Escherichia coli* and *Proteus mirabilis*. Carbenicillin is used mainly for urinary tract infections caused by indole-positive proteus and *Pseudomonas aeruginosa*. Ticarcillin and pipracillin are also indicated for *Pseudomonas* infections plus indole-positive *Proteus* species.

Side and Adverse Effects. The major concern with the use of penicillins is the development of an allergic or hypersensitivity reaction. It is estimated that about 1 to 5 percent of the population has a true allergy to these agents. An allergic reaction can occur in one of three ways: immediate, accelerated, and delayed. The immediate reaction occurs within 2 to 30 minutes after the drug is administered. This reaction may either be a localized one or a systemic anaphylactic reaction. Signs and symptoms associated with the immediate reaction are itchy palms, generalized pruritus or urticaria, feeling of uneasiness, anaphylactic shock (laryngospasm, bronchospasm, hypotension, circulatory collapse), increased capillary permeability, and vasodilation with edema of the mouth, tongue, pharynx, and larynx. The accelerated reaction occurs within 72 hours and is characterized by fever, malaise, and urticaria. The delayed reaction occurs after 72 hours and consists of serum sickness and a variety of skin eruptions.

Another undesirable effect is electrolyte imbalance, which includes hypernatremia, hyperkalemia, or hypokalemia depending on the salt form used. Penicillin may cause local inflammation or abscess when given IM or phlebitis when given IV.

The use of penicillins is also associated with a condition known as superinfection, which is associated with the use of most antibiotics. Superinfection develops when the normal body flora is destroyed, altering the normal pH. This allows the overgrowth of yeast (*Candida*) and gram-negative bacteria.

Toxic accumulation of the penicillins can occur with decreased renal function. Reactions to toxic blood levels of penicillins are bone marrow depression and neuromuscular irritation (muscle twitching, lethargy, seizures, and coma).

Contraindications and Cautions. The use of a penicillin is contraindicated in any individual with a known penicillin allergy. Cautious use of a penicillin in those individuals with a known cephalosporin allergy or with a history of other hypersensitivity reactions. Cautious use in those with decreased renal function, neuromuscular diseases, and in neonates, infants, the elderly, and mothers who are breast feeding.

NURSING IMPLICATIONS

- It is essential for the nurse to take a good drug and medical history of the patient. Any report of a previous allergic reaction to a penicillin derivative precludes the use of a penicillin, except in extreme cases and under very close medical supervision. A past history of an allergic reaction to a cephalosporin indicates the possibility of a cross-reaction and the patient should be closely observed by the nurse. If the patient has a history of cardiovascular disease (e.g., hypertension, congestive heart failure), the nurse should be especially attentive in monitoring the patient for signs of a worsening condition.
- The nurse should monitor laboratory values for electrolyte imbalance paying particular attention to sodium and potassium levels. Normal plasma concentration for adults is 3.5 to 5 mEq/L. This is especially important for patients with cardiovascular problems and for those on a digitalis preparation. Ticarcillin and piperacillin are associated with a higher incidence of potassium depletion.
- If cultures have been ordered, it is important that the nurse ensure that the samples are taken prior to the administration of the first dose of the antibiotic.
- For maximum absorption, oral medications should be administered on an empty stomach 1 hour before and 2 hours after meals with a full glass of water.
- Penicillins have a short half-life ($t_{1/2}$); therefore, they should be administered at fixed intervals around the clock to ensure adequate blood levels throughout the 24-hour period.
- For parenteral administration of penicillins, there are precautions for the nurse to observe. Intravenous infusions are irritating to the veins and cause phlebitis; therefore, the IV site should be inspected frequently. IM injections should be deep into a large muscle mass. Accidental injection near or in a nerve can cause great pain and injury. The IM injection itself can be painful and may be ordered to be given with either 1 or 2 percent lidocaine. Great care should be taken by the nurse not to accidently inject a repository preparation into a vein, which can lead to circulatory collapse and death.
- After administering a dose of penicillin, the nurse should observe the patient for 30 minutes in case an allergic reaction occurs. The nurse should also be prepared to take the appropriate action if a reaction does occur.
- Oral administration of penicillins is associated with nausea, vomiting, diarrhea, and gastrointestinal upset.
- The nurse should assess the patient for signs of improvement.
- Ampicillin is associated with a higher incidence of diarrhea and skin rashes. Ampicillin also decreases the effectiveness of birth control tablets. Patients should be warned of this effect.
- Penicillin should not be used with bacteriostatic antibiotics such as erythromycin, tetracyclines, and chloramphenicol. An exception is the concomitant use of a penicillin with an aminoglycoside. The use of these antibiotics in combination appears to have a synergistic effect.
- Simultaneous administration of probenicid or sulfinpyrazone decreases renal excretion of penicillin causing an accumulation of the drug, which causes higher and prolonged blood levels of the antibiotic.
- In order to maximize efficiency against penicillinase-producing bacteria, amox-

icillin (as Augmentin) and ticarcillin (as Timentin) have been formulated with potassium clavulate, a compound that inactivates penicillinase.
- Most penicillins are administered every 4 to 6 hours depending on the severity of the infection. Amoxicillin, because of its high absorption, may be dosed every 8 hours.
- Signs and symptoms of superinfection caused by *Candida* overgrowth include diarrhea, vaginal discharge, sore mouth, and black furry tongue.

Cephalosporins

The cephalosporins were first isolated in 1948 from the fungus *Cephalosporium acremonium*, which was found near the sewage outlet in Cagliori, Sardinia. The antibiotic secreted by this fungus was found to have a broad spectrum of antibiotic activity.

The cephalosporins are classified according to generations (Table 16–2). This system is based on the drug's spectrum of activity against both gram-positive and gram-negative bacteria. The first generation cephalosporins inhibit many gram-positive and gram-negative bacteria with little advantage over the penicillins except for *Klebsiella* infections. The second generation cephalosporins offer little advantage over the first with respect to gram-positive bacteria; however, they do possess a greater spectrum of activity against gram-negative bacteria. The third generation agents have an even greater spectrum of activity against gram-negative bacteria, including *Pseudomonas* and *Bacteroides fragilis*. In addition, the third generation agents also penetrate the blood–brain barrier to a greater extent than the agents of the first and second generations, making them useful in certain cases of meningitis.

TABLE 16–2. CEPHALOSPORINS GROUPED ACCORDING TO GENERATION

Generic Name	Trade Name(s)	Route(s) of Administration
Parenteral agents		
First generation		
cefazolin	Ancef	IM, IV
	Kefzol	
cephalothin	Keflin	IM, IV
	Seffin	
cephapirin	Cefadyl	IM, IV
cephradine	Anspor	IM, IV
	Velosef	
Second generation		
cefamandole	Mandol	IM, IV
cefonicid	Monocid	IM, IV
ceforanide	Precef	IM, IV
cefoxitin	Mefoxin	IM, IV
cefuroxime	Zinacef	IM, IV
Third generation		
cefoperazone	Cefobid	IM, IV
cefotaxime	Claforan	IM, IV
cetizoxime	Cefizox	IM, IV
moxalactam	Moxam	IM, IV
Oral agents		
cefaclor	Ceclor	PO
cefadroxil	Duricef	PO
	Ultracef	
cephalexin	Keflex	PO
cephradine	Anspor	PO
	Velosef	

With time, organisms that are resistant to the cephalosporins have emerged. The resistance that has developed is similar to the one described for the penicillins, i.e., the bacteria produce enzymes, which are known as beta-lactamases. The first and second generation cephalosporins are more susceptible to this enzymatic attack than the third generation agents.

Action and Fate. The cephalosporins inhibit cell wall synthesis in susceptible bacteria in a way similar to the penicillins. Also, like the penicillins they are bactericidal.

They are excreted unchanged via the urine by both glomerular filtration and renal tubular secretion. The cephalosporins will cross the placenta and are found in breast milk.

Uses. The cephalosporins are broad-spectrum antibiotics. The first and second generation agents are not considered agents of choice for any bacterial infection. They are frequently used to decrease the incidence of infections associated with certain surgical procedures, to treat uncomplicated urinary tract infections, and to treat infections of the respiratory tract.

The third generation cephalosporins have been used to treat meningitis caused by *Escherichia coli*, *Klebsiella*, *Proteus*, and *Hemophilia influenza*.

Side and Adverse Effects. The cephalosporins can cause allergic reactions such as skin rash, fever, urticaria, and anaphylaxis. Diarrhea, nausea, vomiting, and anorexia may also occur.

All the cephalosporins are potentially nephrotoxic and may cause transient elevations in serum creatinine and blood urea nitrogen (BUN) values. If used within recommended doses, however, the cephalosporins available today rarely cause renal damage.

Superinfection frequently occurs with cephalosporins with *Candida* being the usual pathogen.

Intravenous infusion of cephalosporins can cause phlebitis and thrombophlebitis. Intramuscular injections are painful and can cause induration or sterile abscess.

There are specific adverse reactions that apply to certain cephalosporins. With moxalactam, excessive bleeding may occur. The exact cause is not known; however, it can be prevented by administering vitamin K to the patient. If alcohol is ingested by the patient while receiving cefamandole, moxalactam, or cefoperazone, a disulfiram or Antabuse reaction (nausea, vomiting, flushing) will occur.

Contraindications and Cautions. The use of a cephalosporin is contraindicated in an individual who has had a prior hypersensitivity reaction with this class of antibiotics. Cephalosporins should be used cautiously in those who have a penicillin allergy and their use avoided if the prior reaction was anaphylactic or urticarial. They should also be used cautiously in those with impaired kidney function.

NURSING IMPLICATIONS

- Several of the nursing implications are similar to those for penicillins. A thorough drug history should be taken, cultures should be taken prior to the first dose of antibiotic administered, and therapeutic blood levels are maintained for most cephalosporins if they are administered around the clock. The newer agents have longer half-lives and may be dosed less frequently.
- The phlebitis and thrombophlebitis associated with intravenous administration of cephalosporins can be minimized if they are administered into a large vein with a small scale needle.

- Intramuscular injections should be rotated and the sites observed for induration or sterile abscess.
- All cephalosporins, except moxalactam, will cause false-positive reactions with the Clinitest, Benedict's reagents, and Fehling's solution urine glucose tests.
- Avoid alcoholic beverages or preparations (e.g., elixirs) in patients who are being treated with cefamandole, moxalactam, and cefoperazone.
- Closely observe patients who are being treated with moxalactam for unexplained bleeding.
- Instruct the patient to report any indication of a superinfection. Early signs include white patches in mouth, black hairy tongue, mucosal erosions, diarrhea, or vaginal discharge.

Tetracyclines

The tetracyclines are a large group of antibiotics and semisynthetic derivatives derived from two species of *Streptomyces* bacteria. The various derivatives offer no therapeutic advantage over one another. The main difference among them is the dose and dosing interval, which is related to the half-life of the individual drug (Table 16–3).

Action and Fate. All the tetracyclines are well absorbed. They exert their antimicrobial action by inhibiting protein synthesis in susceptible bacteria.

All the tetracyclines concentrate in the liver, but the extent of hepatic metabolism is unknown. Excretion is primarily by glomerular filtration via the urine. Tetracyclines cross the placenta and enter breast milk.

TABLE 16–3. TETRACYCLINES

Generic Name	Trade Name(s)	Half-life ($t_{1/2}$) (hr)	Dosage Form(s) and Route(s) of Administration	Dosing
chlortetracycline HCl	Aureomycin	5.6–7	Oral caps; parenteral (IV)	Oral: 250–500 mg qid IV: 250–500 mg q6–12h NTE[a] 500 mg q6h
tetracycline HCl	Achromycin V Robitet Sumycin	6–12	Oral caps; parenteral (IV)	Oral: 250–500 mg qid IV: 250–500 mg q12h NTE[a] 500 mg q6h
oxytetracycline HCl	Terramycin	6–10	Oral caps; parenteral (IV)	Oral: 250–500 mg qid IV: 250–500 mg q12h NTE[a] 500 mg q6h
methacycline HCl	Rondomycin	7–15	Oral caps	Oral: 150 mg qid or 300 mg bid
demeclocycline HCl	Declomycin	10–17	Oral caps and tabs	Oral: 150 mg qid or 300 mg bid
minocycline HCl	Minocin	11–26	Oral caps; parenteral (IV)	Oral: 200 mg stat, then 100 mg bid IV: 200 mg, then 100 mg q12h NTE[a] 400 mg qd
doxycycline HCl	Vibramycin	14–24	Oral caps and tabs; parenteral (IV)	Oral: 100 mg bid for 1 day then 100 mg qd IV: 200 mg for 1 dose, then 100 to 200 mg qd in 1 or 2 doses

[a] NTE = not to exceed

Uses. The tetracyclines are broad-spectrum antibiotics with a variety of uses. They may be used for many gram-positive and gram-negative infections, and they are considered drugs of choice for brucellosis, cholera, and relapsing fever. They are also alternative drugs of choice for rickettsial infections such as Rocky Mountain spotted fever (with chloramphenicol) and *Mycoplasma* pneumonia (with erythromycin). The tetracyclines are also effective in treating *Neisseria gonorrhoeae* and may be used as an alternative for those who are allergic to penicillin. Tetracycline is also used to treat inflammatory acne.

Side and Adverse Effects. Side effects are common with the tetracyclines, but they are not usually serious. Gastrointestinal upset is the major side effect. This includes anorexia, heartburn, nausea, vomiting, diarrhea, and flatulence.

Tetracyclines tend to bind or complex with calcium. In adults they may deposit in teeth causing a yellow-brown discoloration. In children younger than 8 years old, this calcium-binding property causes tooth malformation (enamel hypoplasia) in addition to tooth discoloration. If tetracyclines are taken during pregnancy, growth retardation or malformation of fetal bones can occur.

Since the tetracyclines are broad-spectrum antibiotics, they can destroy normal body flora causing an overgrowth of pathogens leading to superinfection.

Photosensitivity occurs with the tetracyclines but to a greater degree with demeclocycline and chlortetracycline. This adverse reaction will cause an individual to become severely sunburned with just a short exposure to the sun.

About 50 percent of the individuals taking minocycline will experience inner ear disturbances (vertigo and ataxia).

Contraindications and Cautions. The use of tetracyclines is contraindicated in pregnant and lactating women. Their use is also contraindicated in children under 8 years of age unless absolutely necessary. Tetracyclines should be used with caution in those with liver and renal impairment and avoided in those with hypersensitivity reactions to tetracyclines.

NURSING IMPLICATIONS

- Obtain a thorough drug history and obtain any cultures needed prior to first dose of antibiotic.
- Tetracyclines are maximally absorbed on an empty stomach.
- Be especially observant of expiration dates. Outdated tetracyclines degrade to nephrotoxic products that can cause a Fanconi-like syndrome characterized by acidosis, nausea, vomiting, and proteinuria. This condition is usually reversible upon discontinuation of the drug, but some fatalities have been reported. Warn outpatients not to save leftover tetracyclines for future use.
- Products that contain divalent cations (e.g., Ca^{++}, Al^{++}, Mg^{++}, Fe^{++}) should be avoided with oral tetracycline administration. Tetracyclines bind to these cations making absorption impossible. Therefore advise patients to avoid dairy products, antacids, and mineral supplements during therapy.
- Advise individuals to avoid direct sunlight during therapy.
- Instruct patients to report symptoms of superinfection. Early signs include white patches in mouth, black hairy tongue, mucosal erosions, diarrhea, or vaginal discharge.
- Instruct patients to report inner ear disturbances (vertigo) if taking minocycline.
- Food or milk does not significantly reduce the systemic absorption of oral doxycycline.

Aminoglycosides

The prototype of aminoglycosides is streptomycin, which was isolated in 1944. This class is composed of antibiotics and semisynthetic derivatives obtained from *Streptomyces* and micromonosporia. The antibiotics formulated are highly water soluble and must be administered parenterally in order to achieve therapeutic blood levels. Aminoglycosides are listed in Table 16–4.

Action and Fate. The aminoglycosides are usually considered to be bactericidal. Their exact mechanism of action is not known, but it is known that they must penetrate bacteria before they are effective. Their antimicrobial action is probably due to the inhibition of protein synthesis.

The aminoglycosides are excreted unchanged by glomerular filtration. They will cross the placenta.

Uses. The use of aminoglycosides is indicated in severe complicated infections. They are effective against a variety of aerobic gram-negative bacteria and some aerobic gram-positive bacteria.

The parenteral preparations are used to treat bacteremias and also pulmonary, intra-abdominal, soft tissue, bone, or complicated urinary tract infections caused by susceptible bacteria. Kanamycin or neomycin may be given orally prior to bowel surgery to suppress the growth of aerobic bacteria locally. Neomycin may be administered either orally or as a retention enema in the management of hepatic coma. Neomycin is usually applied topically for infections of the eye, ear, or skin.

Side and Adverse Effects. The most serious adverse effects of the aminoglycosides are nephrotoxicity and ototoxicity. The ototoxicity presents as dizziness, vertigo, ataxia, tinnitus, and hearing impairment. The nephrotoxicity that occurs causes an increase in BUN and serum creatinine values and a decrease in creatinine clearance. Cells or casts may also be observed in the urine in addition to protein. The nephrotoxicity caused by aminoglycosides rarely causes oliguria.

The aminoglycosides can also cause neuromuscular blockade, which may on occasion result in respiratory paralysis.

Contraindications and Cautions. The use of aminoglycosides is contraindicated in those with known hypersensitivity reaction to this class of antibiotics. Their use with other nephrotoxic and ototoxic drugs is also contraindicated. Patients with myasthenia gravis should not be treated with these antibiotics. The aminoglycosides should be used cautiously in the elderly, infants, children, and individuals with renal impairment.

TABLE 16–4. AMINOGLYCOSIDES

Generic Name	Trade Name(s)	Dosage Form(s) and Route(s) of Administration
streptomycin	—	Parenteral (IM)
gentamicin	Garamycin	Parenteral (IV, IM); topical cream and ointment; ophthalmic solution and ointment
tobramycin	Nebcin Tobrex	Parenteral (IV, IM); ophthalmic solution
amikacin	Amikin	Parenteral (IV, IM)
kanamycin	Kantrex	Parenteral (IV, IM), oral caps
neomycin	Mycifradin	Parenteral (IM); oral tabs; topical cream and ointment

NURSING IMPLICATIONS

- Obtain a thorough drug and medical history to determine if the patient has had prior hypersensitivity reactions to an aminoglycoside. Determine if patient has myasthenia gravis.
- Obtain cultures prior to first dose.
- Baseline kidney and auditory tests should be obtained with periodic monitoring during treatment period.
- Peak blood level samples are usually drawn 30 minutes post-infusion of an aminoglucoside.
- Observe patient for signs of ototoxicity; monitor laboratory tests for nephrotoxicity.
- Systemic absorption can occur with oral administration; therefore, patient should be monitored for adverse effects.
- Possible additive nephrotoxicity may occur if aminoglycosides are given with cephalosporins. The loop diuretics furosemide and ethacrynic acid may also enhance nephrotoxicity and ototoxicity. Aminoglycosides should not be used with drugs that cause neuromuscular blockade (succinylcholine, tubocurarine, and other related agents used during surgical anesthesia) because of the neuromuscular blockade these antibiotics can cause.
- A synergistic antibacterial effect has been noted when an aminoglycoside is used with a penicillin, principally ticarcillin or pipracillin.

Sulfonamides and Trimethoprim

The agents that comprise the sulfonamide group of anti-infectives are synthetic chemicals that structurally resemble para-aminobenzoic acid (PABA), a component essential in bacterial metabolism (Table 16–5). The sulfonamides were widely available prior to the introduction of the penicillins. They first became available for general use in the early 1930s with the introduction of sulfanilamide. At the present time, their use has declined due partly to the emergence of resistant strains of bacteria and partly to the development of more effective agents. Nevertheless, the sulfonamides still play an important role in the treatment of acute uncomplicated urinary tract infections and some selected systemic infections.

Although trimethoprim is not related to the sulfonamides, its mechanism of action and uses are closely related to the sulfonamides. For these reasons it is included in this section.

Action and Fate. The sulfonamides are bacteriostatic anti-infective agents. In susceptible bacteria, they inhibit the synthesis of folic acid, which is necessary for growth in bacteria, by blocking the enzymatic conversion of PABA to folic acid (Fig. 16–1). The sulfonamides are all metabolized in the liver. Active drug and metabolites are excreted via the urine by glomerular filtration. They easily cross the placenta and are found in breast milk.

Trimethoprim is primarily a bactericidal agent. It also blocks the synthesis of folic acid but at another site in the pathway (Fig. 16–1). A portion of trimethoprim is metabolized in the liver and then both metabolite and active drug are excreted in the urine via glomerular filtration and tubular secretion. It easily crosses the placenta and is found in breast milk.

Uses. The most important use of the sulfonamides is for the treatment of acute, uncomplicated urinary tract infections caused by *Escherichia coli*, *Klebsiella*, *Proteus mirabilis*, and *Proteus vulgaris*. They may also be used for chlamydial infections

TABLE 16–5. SULFONAMIDES AND TRIMETHOPRIM

Generic Name	Trade Name(s)	Dosage Form(s) and Route(s) of Administration	Indication of Use
sulfamethizole	Thiosulfil	Oral tabs	Urinary tract infections
sulfamethoxazole[a]	Gantanol	Oral tabs	Urinary tract and specific systemic infections
sulfasalazine	Azulfidine	Oral tabs	Ulcerative colitis and regional enteritis
sulfisoxazole[b]	Gantrisin	Oral tabs; parenteral (IV, IM, SQ) vaginal cream; ophthalmic solution and ointment	Urinary tract and specific systemic infections, vaginitis, and superficial ocular infection
mafenide acetate	Sulfamylon	Topical cream	Prevention and treatment of infection in second and third degree burns
silver sulfadiazine	Silvadene	Topical cream	Same as mefanide
sulfacetamide	Bleph-10 Sodium Sulamyd	Ophthalmic solution and ointment; scalp and skin lotion	Superficial ocular infection and various dermatologic conditions
sulfamethoxazole/ trimethoprim (cotrimoxazole)	Bactrim Septra	Oral tabs and parenteral (IV)	Urinary tract and specific systemic infections
trimethoprim	Priloprim Trimpex	Oral tabs	Urinary tract infection

[a] Sulfamethoxazole with phenazopyridine = Azo-Gantrisin.
[b] Sulfisoxazole with phenazopyridine = Azo-Gantanol.

and for bacillary dysentery caused by some strains of *Shigella*. One sulfonamide, sulfasalazine, is indicated solely for the treatment of mild to moderate ulcerative colitis.

Trimethoprim is recommended for acute, uncomplicated urinary tract infections caused by *E. coli*, *P. mirabalis*, and *Klebsiella*.

Side and Adverse Effects. Most commonly, individuals taking sulfonamides will experience nausea, vomiting, and anorexia. Hypersensitivity reactions are relatively common. Most often these reactions involve the skin and mucous membranes and include skin rashes, urticaria, and photosensitivity.

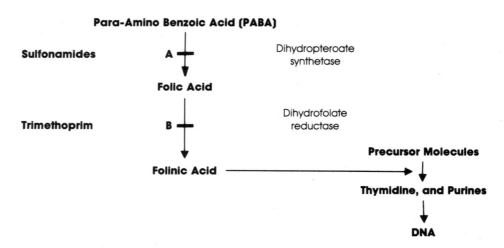

Figure 16–1. Diagrammatic representation of the site of enzymatic blockade of most sulfonamides (**A**) and trimethoprim (**B**) in the inhibition of DNA synthesis in susceptible bacteria.

Kidney damage was a real danger with the sulfonamides that were first available for general use. The early agents tended to crystallize in the acidic pH of the urine (crystalluria). The risk of kidney damage with the newer agents is greatly reduced because of their greater water solubility.

With trimethoprim, one most frequently sees rash, pruritis, and gastrointestinal upsets which include nausea, vomiting, and epigastric upset.

Contraindications and Cautions. The sulfonamides should be used with caution in individuals with impaired renal function. Their use is contraindicated in those who have a history of prior hypersensitivity reactions.

Sulfonamides displace bilirubin from plasma protein-binding sites causing an increase in free bilirubin. In the fetus or neonate, this free bilirubin will penetrate the immature blood–brain barrier causing neurological damage (a condition known as kernicterus). For this reason sulfonamides are contraindicated in pregnant or lactating women and neonates.

Trimethoprim should be used with caution in individuals with impaired renal function.

NURSING IMPLICATIONS

Sulfonamides

- Obtain a drug history for previous allergic reaction to a sulfonamide. Ascertain if patient is pregnant.
- Take specimen for culture prior to first dose. For a urine culture this would involve a clean catch specimen.
- Advise the patient to avoid urine-acidifying substances such as vitamin C and cranberry juice while taking a sulfonamide and to increase water intake to 1200 ml a day while taking a sulfonamide.
- Instruct the patient to report any rash that appears.
- The gastrointestinal upset may be reduced by taking the medication with meals.
- Advise the patient to avoid unnecessary exposure to the sun.

Trimethoprim

- Advise patient to report the appearance of a rash or pruritis.
- Gastrointestinal upsets may be reduced with food.

Trimethoprim and Sulfamethoxazole (Bactrim, Septra)

Action and Fate. Antibacterial synergism occurs when these two anti-infective agents are formulated into a single preparation. In addition, fewer resistant organisms develop because each agent inhibits a different step in the synthesis of folic acid.

Uses. The use of this combination is indicated for a number of infections: urinary tract infections, acute otitis media, acute chronic bronchitis, shigellosis, and *Pneumocystis carinii*.

Contraindications and Cautions. For contraindications and cautions, please refer to individual agents.

NURSING IMPLICATIONS

For nursing implications, please refer to the individual agents.

Urinary Tract Antiseptics and Phenazopyridine

This class of drugs contains a number of structurally unrelated agents. For this reason each agent will be considered individually.

The anti-infective agents listed in Table 16–6 are used for only one indication: the treatment of uncomplicated urinary tract infections. They are effective because they are excreted in the urine in their active form. Additional advantages that make these drugs important and useful in the management of recurrent or chronic urinary tract infection are that they are relatively nontoxic and that bacteria rarely develop resistance to these agents.

Phenazopyridine is also included with this group even though it is not an antibacterial agent but an analgesic used to relieve the dysuria that frequently accompanies a urinary tract infection.

Methenamine Hippurate or Mandelate

Action and Fate. Methenamine itself has no antibacterial activity. Its action results from the release of formaldehyde in an acid solution. It is the formaldehyde that destroys bacteria by denaturing bacterial proteins. The drug is primarily excreted unchanged in the urine.

Uses. Methenamine is active against a variety of gram-positive and gram-negative bacteria. It is mainly used for prophylactic therapy in individuals with chronic recurring urinary tract infections.

Side and Adverse Effects. This agent is relatively safe and well tolerated by most individuals. It may cause some nausea, gastric distress, rash, and dysuria.

Contraindications and Cautions. The use of methenamine is contraindicated with sulfonamides, and in individuals with impaired renal function or hepatic disease.

NURSING IMPLICATIONS

- Gastric irritation may be minimized if given with food or milk.
- The nurse should monitor or teach the patient to monitor urine pH with nitrazine paper. A pH of 5.5 or below is needed in order to maintain an adequate concentration for antibacterial action. Vitamin C is usually ordered with methenamine in order to acidify the urine.
- Urine culture and sensitivity tests should be done prior to initiation of treatment. Instruct the patient how to obtain a clean catch specimen.

TABLE 16–6. URINARY TRACT ANTI-INFECTIVE AGENTS AND PHENAZOPYRIDINE

Generic Name	Trade Name(s)	Route(s) of Administration	Major Use
methenamine hippurate	Hiprex Urex	PO	Urinary tract infections
methenamine mandelate	Mandelamine	PO	Urinary tract infections
nalidixic acid	NegGram	PO	Urinary tract infections
nitrofurantoin	Furadantin	PO	Urinary tract infections
nitrofurantoin (macrocrystals)	Macrodantin	PO, IV, IM	Urinary tract infections
phenazopyridine	Pyridium	PO	Relief of pain associated with dysuria

Nalidixic Acid

Action and Fate. The antibacterial action of nalidixic acid appears to be related to the inhibition of DNA synthesis in susceptible bacteria.

Most of the drug is metabolized in the liver and excreted as an active metabolite, an inactive metabolite, and active drug. The drug crosses the placenta and a small amount is found in breast milk.

Uses. Nalidixic acid has a rather narrow spectrum of activity. It is most effective in treating urinary tract infections caused by the majority of *Proteus* strains, *Klebsiella,* and *E. coli.*

Side and Adverse Effects. Most commonly patients complain of nausea, vomiting, abdominal pain, and diarrhea. There are also central nervous system effects such as drowsiness, dizziness, and vertigo.

Contraindications and Cautions. The use of nalidixic acid is contraindicated in pregnant women and individuals with a history of convulsive disorders. The drug should be used cautiously in those with impaired renal or liver function.

NURSING IMPLICATIONS

- Urine culture and sensitivity tests should be done prior to initiation of treatment. Instruct the patient how to obtain a clean catch specimen.
- May be administered with food or milk to minimize gastrointestinal distress.

Nitrofurantoin

Action and Fate. Nitrofurantoin is available in both oral and parenteral forms. It appears to act by inhibiting several enzyme systems in susceptible bacteria, but the exact mechanism by which this occurs is unknown.

About 60 percent of the drug is rapidly metabolized in the liver; the remainder is excreted unchanged in the urine. The drug crosses the placenta, and it is also found in breast milk.

Use. Nitrofurantoin is effective in the treatment of uncomplicated urinary tract infections. Its spectrum of activity is wide and includes both gram-positive and gram-negative bacteria.

Side and Adverse Effects. Most individuals treated with nitrofurantoin will experience nausea, vomiting, diarrhea, abdominal pain, and fever.

Contraindications and Cautions. Nitrofurantoin is contraindicated in individuals with anuria, oliguria, and significant impaired renal function.

NURSING IMPLICATIONS

- Nitrofurantoin should be administered with food or milk to minimize gastrointestinal irritation and to enhance absorption.
- Urine culture and sensitive tests should be done prior to initiation of treatment. Instruct the patient how to obtain a clean catch specimen.
- Monitor patient input–output ratio. The drug should be discontinued if oliguria occurs.

Phenazopyridine

Action and Fate. Phenazopyridine is not an anti-infective agent. It has an analgesic effect on the bladder mucosa, which relieves the pain, burning, and urgency associated with urinary tract infections. Phenazopyridine is available as a single entity tablet or in combination with a sulfonamide.

The drug is partially metabolized in the liver and is excreted both as metabolite and unchanged drug. It may cross the placenta.

Use. Phenazopyridine is used for symptomatic relief of dysuria associated with infections, trauma, surgery, or instrumentation.

Side and Adverse Effects. Side effects with phenazopyridine are infrequent. The patient may complain of gastrointestinal distress, headache, and vertigo.

Contraindications and Cautions. Phenazopyridine should not be used in individuals with renal insufficiency, glomerulonephritis, or pyelonephritis, and it should not be used during pregnancy.

NURSING IMPLICATIONS

- Phenazopyridine may be administered with food to minimize gastrointestinal distress.
- Advise the patient that the drug will cause a red-orange color change of the urine, which can stain undergarments.
- The drug should be discontinued as soon as the dysuria is relieved.

Miscellaneous Anti-infective Agents

Included in this group of miscellaneous agents are chloramphenicol, the macrolides, lincosamides, and metronidazole. Since each is unrelated, they will be considered separately.

Chloramphenicol

Chloramphenicol is the only available agent of this type. It is a naturally occurring antibiotic produced by the organism *Streptomyces venezuelae*. It is usually bacteriostatic, but may be bactericidal against *H. influenzae* and *B. fragilis* at higher concentrations.

Action and Fate. Chloramphenicol is thought to inhibit bacterial growth by interfering with protein synthesis. Chloramphenicol undergoes conjugation with glucuronic acid in the liver and then is rapidly excreted in the urine. It easily crosses the placenta and it also appears in breast milk.

Uses. Chloramphenicol is effective against a variety of gram-negative and gram-positive bacteria and most anaerobic microorganisms. Despite its broad and effective spectrum of activity, chloramphenicol is held in reserve for serious life-threatening infections that do not respond to less toxic agents.

It is very effective in the treatment of acute typhoid fever and other *Salmonella* infections. Chloramphenicol easily penetrates the blood–brain barrier and therefore is useful in treating infections of the central nervous system caused by susceptible organisms. It is considered to be one of the drugs of choice (with ampicillin) for meningitis caused by *H. influenzae*. It is the alternative drug of choice for Rocky Mountain spotted fever in cases in which tetracyclines are contraindicated.

Side and Adverse Effects. With the use of this antibiotic, the major concern is the occurrence of one of two types of bone marrow depression. The first type, which is a true toxic reaction, is dose related and is reversible when the drug is discontinued. The other is nondose related and irreversible and may occur after a

TABLE 16–7. MISCELLANEOUS ANTI-INFECTIVE AGENTS

Generic Name	Trade Name(s)	Dosage Form(s) and Route(s) of Administration
Miscellaneous antibiotics		
chloramphenicol	Chloromycetin chloroptic Econochlor Mychel	Oral caps; parenteral (IV); ophthalmic ointment and solution; otic solution
chloramphenicol palmitate	Chloromycetin palmitate	Oral suspension
chloramphenicol sodium succinate	Mychel-S	Parenteral (IV)
erythromycin base	Eryc E-Mycin Ilotycin	Oral tabs; ophthalmic ointment
erythromycin estolate	Ilosone	Oral caps and suspension
erythromycin ethylsuccinate	E.E.S. Erythrocin Pediamycin	Oral tabs and suspension; parenteral (IV)
erythromycin gluceptate	Ilotycin Gluceptate	Parenteral (IV)
erythromycin lactobionate	Erythrocin Lactobionate	Parenteral (IV)
erythromycin stearate	Erypar Erythrocin Stearate	Oral tabs
clindamycin hydrochloride	Cleocin	Oral caps
clindamycin palmitate hydrochloride	Cleocin Pediatric	Oral suspension
clindamycin phosphate	Cleocin Cleocin T	Parenteral (IV, IM); topical solution
lincomycin hydrochloride	Lincocin	Oral caps and syrup; parenteral (IV, IM)
Antitrichomonal agent		
Metronidazole	Flagyl	Oral tabs and parenteral (IV)

single dose or weeks or months after the initial treatment time. This irreversible bone marrow depression can cause pancytopenia, agranulocytosis, aplastic anemia, and leukemia. It is often fatal.

Other side effects associated with chloramphenicol are nausea, vomiting, diarrhea, headache, and hypersensitivity reactions.

An adverse effect associated with the use of chloramphenicol in premature infants and neonates under 2 weeks of age is the gray syndrome. It is due to the immaturity of the liver enzyme system in premature infants and neonates, which in turn causes toxic accumulation of the drugs. The symptoms of this reaction include abdominal distention, pallied cyanosis, flaccidity, irregular respiration, acute circulatory failure, and death.

Contraindications and Cautions. Chloramphenicol is contraindicated for minor infections, prophylactic treatment, or therapy with other drugs that also cause bone marrow depression. It should be used cautiously in individuals with liver or kidney impairment, and premature and full-term infants.

NURSING IMPLICATIONS

- Patients treated with chloramphenicol usually require hospitalization.
- It is important for the nurse to closely observe and note signs and symptoms of bone marrow depression, and to closely monitor blood test results for leukopenia, thrombocytopenia, and reticulocytosis.
- The nondose-related toxicity associated with chloramphenicol may appear weeks or months after therapy. Counsel patient to report any bruising, bleeding, fatigue, or unexplained fever promptly.
- Closely observe prematures and newborns for the gray syndrome. Promptly report any signs or symptoms.

Macrolides

Only one agent in this group, erythromycin, will be discussed. Erythromycin was isolated in the early 1950s from the metabolic products of the bacteria *Strepto-*

myces erythreus. It is considered to be one of the safest antibiotics in use today. It is also considered to be the safe alternative for pen G or pen VK in individuals with penicillin allergy because of its similar antibacterial spectrum of activity.

Action and Fate. Erythromycin acts by inhibiting protein synthesis in susceptible bacteria. It may exert bacteriostatic or bactericidal action, depending on the organism and drug concentration.

The oral forms of erythromycin exist in various salt forms and formulations in order to enhance absorption and minimize inactivation by gastric acid.

Erythromycin concentrates in the liver and is excreted unchanged in the bile and feces. It crosses the placenta and is excreted in breast milk.

Uses. Erythromycin may be used to treat mild to moderate gram-positive infections of the skin, soft tissue, and body cavities. It is the drug of choice for *Legionella pneumophila* (Legionnaire's disease) and an alternative drug of choice with tetracycline for primary atypical pneumonia caused by *Mycoplasma pneumoniae*. It is also used for acute pelvic inflammatory disease caused by *Neisseria gonorrhoeae* and for primary syphilis in those with penicillin allergies.

Erythromycin base is used with neomycin prior to surgery for bowel sterilization. The ophthalmic ointment is indicated for the prophylaxis (in newborns) of ophthalmia neonatorum caused by *N. gonorrhoeae* or *Chlamydia trachomatis*.

Side and Adverse Effects. Erythromycin is seldom associated with any serious adverse effect. Orally, the drug does cause nausea, vomiting, heartburn, indigestion, and diarrhea.

A serious adverse effect associated with the estolate salt of erythromycin is cholestatic hepatitis, a hypersensitivity reaction. Symptoms include right upper quandrant pain or tenderness, jaundice, fever, malaise, nausea, and vomiting.

Contraindications and Cautions: Erythromycin is contraindicated in any individual with prior hypersensitivity reaction. It should be used cautiously in those with impaired liver function.

NURSING IMPLICATIONS

- Erythromycin should be taken on an empty stomach to ensure maximum absorption. If gastrointestinal symptoms persist, however, food or snack may be given with the medication.
- Instruct the patient to report signs of superinfection. Early signs include white patches in mouth, black hairy tongue, mucosal erosions, diarrhea, or vaginal discharge.
- Closely observe patients for liver dysfunction especially with erythromycin estolate.

Lincosamides

There are two antibiotics in this class: lincomycin and clindamycin. Lincomycin is the prototype. It is produced by the bacteria *Streptomyces lincolnensis*. Its use is limited at this time. It has been replaced by its semisynthetic derivative, clindamycin, which is better absorbed after oral administration, more effective, and less toxic. For this reason the discussion will primarily focus on clindamycin.

Action and Fate. Both antibiotics inhibit protein synthesis in susceptible bacteria. The agents are primarily bacteriostatic but may be bactericidal depending on the organism and concentration of the drug.

Both agents are metabolized in the liver to both active and inactive metabolites, which are then excreted via the urine, bile, and feces. Both cross the placenta and both may appear in breast milk.

Uses. Neither drug is considered to be a first line antibiotic because of the potentially fatal pseudomembraneous colitis that can occur (see Side and Adverse Effects). Clindamycin is effective against susceptible strains of anaerobic bacteria especially *Bacteroides fragilis*. Its use is also indicated in infections caused by susceptible aerobic gram-positive bacteria resistant to both penicillin and erythromycin. Clindamycin, used topically as a solution, has been found to be very effective in the treatment of acne vulgaris.

Lincomycin offers no therapeutic advantage over clindamycin.

Side and Adverse Effects. The most frequent side effect reported is diarrhea. In addition, the lincosamides can cause pseudomembraneous colitis, a potentially fatal condition. This intestinal disorder is caused by an overgrowth of *Clostridium difficile*, a bacterium that is resistant to both agents. It is the toxic byproduct secreted by this organism that causes the ulceration of the intestinal mucosa.

Other mild hypersensitivity reactions reported for both agents are pruritis, rash, and urticaria.

Contraindications and Cautions. The use of either of these drugs is contraindicated in individuals with a prior hypersensitivity reaction and in individuals with a history of regional enteritis or ulcerative colitis.

NURSING IMPLICATIONS

- It is important for the nurse to ascertain from the patient if there has been any history of colitis.
- It is important for the nurse to differentiate between diarrhea caused by gastric irritation and diarrhea caused by the pseudomembraneous colitis. The latter may have blood and mucus present.
- Oral vancomycin or cholestyramine has been used to treat the pseudomembraneous colitis caused by *Clostridium difficile*.
- The topical application of clindamycin for acne has not been associated with the development of any systemic adverse effects.

Metronidazole

Metronidazole is a synthetic agent with both antibacterial and antiprotozoan properties.

Action and Fate. This agent can be described as bactericidal, amebecidal, and trichomonacidal. The exact mechanism of action is not known. Metronidazole is metabolized in the liver and excreted in the urine. It easily crosses the placenta and is distributed into breast milk.

Uses. Metronidazole has a number of uses. It is used orally in the treatment of symptomatic and asymptomatic trichomonasis in men and women. It is used orally in the treatment of acute intestinal amebiasis and amebic liver abscess caused by *Entamoeba histolytica*. For serious anaerobic bacterial infections, metronidazole may be used either orally or intravenously.

Side and Adverse Effects. The most usual side effects experienced are nausea, vomiting, gastrointestinal upset, diarrhea, and headache. The drug can also cause a metallic taste in the mouth. A reddish-brown color change in urine may also be noted. A disulfiram (Antabuse) effect will occur if any type of alcoholic preparation is consumed during therapy.

Contraindications and Cautions. Use of the drug is not recommended during the first trimester of pregnancy, in nursing mothers, and in individuals with active central nervous system disease or blood dyscrasias.

NURSING IMPLICATIONS

- Administer metronidazole with food to minimize gastrointestinal upset.
- Oral dosing regimens for trichomonas may be individualized depending on the expected compliance. There are two commonly employed schemes. One regimen requires three times a day for 7 days; the other is giving a total dose of 250 mg as one or two doses.
- All sexual partners should receive concurrent treatment and the individuals should abstain from sexual activity during treatment.
- Warn the individual not to drink alcoholic beverages during treatment to avoid antabuse effect (intense flushing, tachycardia, nausea, vomiting, and circulatory collapse).
- Therapy should be discontinued if any central nervous system side effects develop.
- Intravenous infusions of metronidazole should not be refrigerated. They should be protected from light, and they should be infused alone.

Antifungal Agents

Two types of antifungal agents will be discussed in this section: those used for systemic fungal infections and those used for nonsystemic infections. Systemic fungal infections are by far the most serious ones and the most difficult to treat. They are caused by a variety of fungal organisms (Table 16–8).

There are two major types of nonsystemic or superficial fungal infections: dermatophytic and mucocutaneous. There are many nonprescription prepara-

TABLE 16–8. ANTIFUNGAL AGENTS

Generic Name	Trade Name(s)	Dosage Form(s) and Route(s) of Administration	Indication of Use
Agents for systemic and nonsystemic infections			
amphotericin B	Fungizone	Parenteral (IV); topical cream; ointment; and lotion	Aspergillosis, blastomycosis, coccidioidomycosis, cryptococcosis, disseminated candidiasis, histoplasmosis, and sporotrichosis. Topically: *Candida*
miconazole	Micatin Monistat Monistat 7	Parenteral (IV); topical cream; vaginal cream and suppository	Coccidioidomycosis, candidiasis, cryptococcosis, paracoccidioidomycosis, Topical: candiasis and various tinea infections
Agents for systemic infections			
flucytosine	Anocobon	Oral caps	Cryptococcosis and candiasis
ketoconazole	Nizoral	Oral tabs	Coccidioidomycosis and paracoccidioidomycosis
Agents for nonsystemic infections			
clotrimazole	Lotrimin Gyne-Lotrimin Mycelex Mycelex-G	Topical cream and solution; vaginal cream and tabs; oral troche	Various tinea infections, and candiasis
griseofulvin	Fulvicin-U/F	Oral tabs	Fungal infection of the hair, skin, or nails caused by various species of *Epidermophton, Microsporum,* and *Trichophyton*
nystatin	Mycostatin Nilstat	Oral tabs and suspension; vaginal tabs; topical cream, ointment and powder	Mucocutaneous infections caused by all species of *Candida*

tions available for the treatment of the dermatophytic type and no attempt will be made to cover these agents in this section. Mucocutaneous infections are primarily caused by *Candida albicans,* an organism that is part of the normal body flora. Under certain circumstances, e.g., antibacterial treatment, the balance of the normal body flora is altered causing pathogenic overgrowth, usually *Candida.*

Amphotericin B

Action and Fate. Amphotericin B is an antibiotic produced by *Streptomyces nodosus.* Its antifungal effect is due to an alteration in membrane permeability that allows essential molecules to leak out. The exact metabolic pathway and route of excretion of amphotericin B is unknown.

Uses. Amphotericin B has a broad spectrum of activity against potentially fatal fungal infections including aspergillosis, blastomycosis, coccidioidomycosis, and disseminated candidiasis.

Side and Adverse Effects. There are many unpleasant and potentially toxic reactions that occur with the intravenous administration of amphotericin B. Acute febrile reactions occur frequently accompanied with chills and shaking. It is nephrotoxic and can cause decreased urine output. Other side effects include hypokalemia, arrhythmias, hypo- or hypertension, nausea, vomiting, anorexia, and diarrhea.

The topical application is not associated with any systemic adverse effects. Only localized side effects such as pruritis, burning, and erythema have been reported.

Contraindications and Cautions. This agent should be used with caution in individuals with impaired renal function, and with the concurrent administration of other nephrotoxic drugs.

NURSING IMPLICATIONS

- Intravenous infusion is given slowly, usually over 6 hours. Amphotericin B must be diluted at a minimum ratio of 1 mg of drug to 10 ml of solution if necessary. A final volume of 500 ml, however, is preferred, even if it exceeds the 1 mg to 10 ml ratio.
- A test dose of amphotericin B may be given to evaluate a patient's response to the drug.
- Amphotericin B is not compatible with solutions containing sodium chloride.
- Solutions should be protected from light.
- Monitor vital signs of patient: temperature, blood pressure, and pulse for an increase.
- Patients should have routine electrolyte and blood tests. Kidney function should also be monitored; input–output ratio should be monitored.
- In order to minimize chills and fever, the patient may be given meperidine, diphenhydramine, or a steroid before and during administration of drug.

Clotrimazole

Action and Fate. Clotrimazole is used topically and vaginally for fungal infections. It acts by altering membrane permeability of the fungal cell allowing the loss of essential cellular molecules. Its systemic absorption is negligible following topical or intravaginal application.

Uses. Clotrimazole is used topically for various dermatophytic infections and vaginally for candidiasis caused by *Candida albicans.*

Side and Adverse Effects. Topical application of the drug is associated with localized stinging, erythema, edema, pruritus, and urticaria. The vaginal application of clotrimazole may cause a burning sensation, itching, rash, and various urinary tract irritations.

Contraindications and Cautions. The use of clotrimazole is contraindicated in individuals with a previous hypersensitivity reaction to the drug.

NURSING IMPLICATIONS

- Teach the individual appropriate hygienic procedures to prevent recurrence of infection.
- Advise females to use protective pads during vaginal use of clotrimazole.

Flucytosine

Action and Fate. Flucytosine is a synthetic antifungal agent. Once it has penetrated the infecting organism, it is metabolized to a nucleic acid analogue, which is thought to be responsible for its antifungal activity. The majority of the drug that is excreted from the body is excreted unchanged.

Uses. Flucytosine is used for serious systemic infections caused by *Cryptococcus* and *Candida*.

Side and Adverse Effects. Flucytosine may cause bone marrow depression, gastrointestinal upset, and alterations in liver function tests.

Contraindications and Cautions. The drug should be used with caution in individuals with impaired renal function, bone marrow depression, and hemotologic disorders.

NURSING IMPLICATIONS

- Blood, kidney, and liver function tests should be performed before and during therapy.
- Dosage adjustments should be made for patients with decreased renal function.

Griseofulvin

Action and Fate. Griseofulvin exerts its antifungal action by arresting the division of fungal cells. The drug becomes bound to new keratin of the skin, hair, and nails. These tissues then become highly resistant to infection.

The drug is metabolized in the liver and excreted primarily as metabolites in the urine.

Use. Griseofulvin is used to treat fungal infections of the hair, skin, and nails that are not responsive to topical treatment.

Side and Adverse Effects. The incidence of side effects is low with griseofulvin. The most common side effect is headache. Other side effects include vertigo, fever, nausea, vomiting, and diarrhea.

Contraindications and Cautions. The use of griseofulvin is contraindicated in individuals with hepatic disease and systemic lupus erythematosus. Use with caution in penicillin-sensitive patients.

NURSING IMPLICATIONS

- Duration of treatment depends on time needed to replace infected tissues with new tissue. Depending on the site of infection, the treatment can last from 2 weeks to 6 months.
- Caution patients to avoid prolonged exposure to the sun to avoid hypersensitivity reaction.

Ketoconazole

Action and Fate. Ketoconazole is thought to interfere with the synthesis of fungal cell membranes. It is metabolized in the liver and excreted via the bile into the intestinal tract.

Uses. Ketoconazole can be used to treat mucocutaneous and systemic fungal infections including candidiasis, coccidioidomycosis, and histoplasmosis.

Side and Adverse Effects. The drug is usually well tolerated. Side effects that might occur include nausea, vomiting, diarrhea, pruritus, and headache.

Contraindications and Cautions. Use during pregnancy is not advised. It should be used with caution in individuals with impaired hepatic function.

NURSING IMPLICATIONS

- For adequate systemic absorption to occur, ketoconazole requires an acid pH. Therefore, it should be given 2 hours before any agent that elevates stomach pH. This includes antacids, cimetidine, ranitidine, or an anticholinergic agent.
- If patient is achlorhydric, it may be necessary to give the drug with a diluted solution of hydrochloric acid.

Miconazole

Action and Fate. The mechanism of action of miconazole is unclear, but it appears to prevent the uptake of essential molecules and to cause alteration in the cell wall structure. The drug undergoes hepatic metabolism and is excreted mainly as inactive metabolites in the urine and feces.

Uses. Topically miconazole is used for various dermatophytic and mucocutaneous infections. Parenteral administration is reserved for serious systemic fungal infections.

Side and Adverse Effects. Rapid intravenous infusion can cause tachycardia and cardiac arrhythmias. Topical application can cause vulvovaginal burning, itching, or irritation.

Contraindications and Cautions. The use of miconazole is contraindicated during the first trimester and used with caution during the second and third trimesters of pregnancy.

NURSING IMPLICATIONS

- For intravaginal use, instruct the patient to insert the applicator of drug high into vagina and to use a protective pad to prevent staining and excessive leakage.

Nystatin

Action and Fate. Nystatin alters the permeability of the cell membrane. This allows essential intracellular molecules to leak out. There is no measurable systemic absorption and therefore when given orally the drug is excreted intact in the feces.

Use. Used to treat fungal infections of the skin and mucous membranes caused by *Candida albicans.*

Side and Adverse Effects. Topical application rarely causes any reaction. Orally, the patient may experience mild nausea, vomiting, and diarrhea.

Contraindications and Cautions. The use of nystatin is contraindicated in individuals with prior hypersensitivity reactions.

NURSING IMPLICATIONS

- Nystatin is available in a variety of dosage forms: oral tablet, vaginal tablet, oral suspension, and topical cream, ointment, and powder.
- Protective padding should be worn when vaginal tablets are used to avoid excessive leakage.
- Instruct patient in proper hygienic procedures to prevent recurrence of infection.
- Recurring vaginal fungal infection may be associated with diabetes, pregnancy, and use of birth control pills.

Antiviral Agents

The treatment of viral infections is less successful than that of other pathogenic organisms. Viruses are simple organisms that consist of a strand of genetic material (DNA or RNA) surrounded by a protein coat. They are considered lifeless until they enter living cells. Once inside the host cells the viral genetic material uses the metabolic apparatus of the host cell to replicate itself. For this reason it has been difficult to develop drugs that will selectively kill viruses without harming the host cells.

Even though most of the antiviral agents share similar mechanisms of action, there are differences among them that warrant discussing each separately.

Acyclovir

Action and Fate. Acyclovir is metabolized to acyclovir triphosphate, which inhibits the enzyme responsible for DNA replication. The drug is excreted unchanged via the urine.

TABLE 16–9. ANTIVIRAL AGENTS

Generic Name	Trade Name(s)	Dosage Form(s)	Uses
acyclovir	Zovirax	Parenteral (IV), topical ointment, oral caps	Herpes simplex types 1 and 2, varicella-zoster
amantadine	Symmetrel	Oral caps	Prevention of influenza, (also for parkinsonism)
idoxuridine	Herplex Stoxil	Ophthalmic solution and ointment	Herpes simplex keratitis
trifluridine	Viroptic	Ophthalmic solution	Herpes simplex keratitis
vidarabine (Ara-A)	Vira-A	Parenteral (IV), and ophthalmic ointment	Herpes simplex keratitis, keratoconjunctivitis, viral encephalitis

Uses. Acyclovir is available as a topical cream, oral capsule, and parenteral form. Its use is indicated to treat herpes simplex types 1 and 2 and varicella-zoster virus infections.

Side and Adverse Effects. No serious adverse effects have been noted. Acyclovir primarily causes local irritations at the infusion site and local burning and stinging with topical application.

Contraindications and Cautions. The parenteral form of the drug should be used with caution in patients with impaired renal function.

NURSING IMPLICATIONS

- Monitor infusion site routinely for signs of irritation.
- Aseptic technique should be used with topical preparation to prevent contamination.

Amantadine

Action and Fate. Amantadine prevents viral infection by preventing viral penetration into the host cell. The mechanism by which this occurs is not known. The drug is not metabolized; it is excreted unchanged in the urine.

Uses. Amantadine is used in high risk individuals prophylactically against influenza A virus. Also used for Parkinson's disease.

Side and Adverse Effects. Central nervous system side effects occur most frequently with amantadine: confusion, lightheadedness, headaches, hallucinations, anxiety, insomnia, psychosis.

Contraindications and Cautions. Amantadine should be used with caution in individuals with hepatic disease, renal impairment, and the elderly with cerebral arteriosclerosis.

NURSING IMPLICATIONS

- As a prophylactic for influenza, amantadine should be started prior to anticipated contact with infected individuals and continued through flu season—usually 5 to 6 weeks.
- Closely monitor individuals with cardiovascular problems.
- Observe individuals for psychic disturbances.

Idoxuridine and Trifluridine

Action and Fate. Both agents are incorporated into the viral DNA during its replication instead of thymidine. This substituted molecule in the DNA causes an increased rate of mutation, erroneous protein synthesis, and a fragile strand of DNA more susceptible to fragmentation.

Neither agent is absorbed systemically in an appreciable amount.

Use. Both agents are used in the eye to treat herpes simplex keratitis.

Side and Adverse Effects. Both agents may cause local irritation, photophobia, and edema of the eyelids. Hypersensitivity reactions have been reported for both agents.

Contraindications and Cautions. Both agents should be used under the supervision of an ophthalmologist. Healing may be delayed with idoxuridine because it also inhibits DNA synthesis in the host cells.

NURSING IMPLICATIONS

- The ophthalmic solution of idoxuridine should be stored in the refrigerator.
- The tip of the eyedropper or the tip of the ointment tube should be kept clean and should not come in contact with the eyelid or lashes.
- The nurse should stress the importance of following the instructions for application exactly and of completing the prescribed course.

Vidarabine (Ara-A)

Action and Fate. Vidarabine appears to inhibit viral replication by blocking DNA replication. Vidarabine and its metabolites are excreted primarily by the kidneys.

Uses. The intravenous form of vidarabine is indicated in the treatment of encephalitis caused by herpes simplex. It is used topically for herpes simplex keratitis and keratoconjunctivitis.

Side and Adverse Effects. Vidarabine usually causes few side effects. Intravenous use is associated with nausea, vomiting, diarrhea, and anorexia. Patients have also experienced dizziness, hallucinations, ataxia, and psychosis. Topical application to the eye may cause burning, irritation, pain, and photophobia.

Contraindications and Cautions. Vidarabine should be used with caution in patients with impaired liver or kidney function.

NURSING IMPLICATIONS

- Parenteral infusions of vidarabine are not refrigerated.
- Intravenous infusions are infused over a 12- to 24-hour period using an inline filter (0.45 μm or smaller). A maximum of 450 mg of vidarabine will dissolve in 1 L of fluid. Therefore, patients should be carefully observed for fluid overload.
- Instruct patients on proper aseptic application techniques for ophthamalogic preparation.

Review Questions

PENICILLINS

1. Superinfection occurs more frequently with:
   a. narrow-spectrum antibiotics
   b. acid-stable antibiotics
   c. parenteral administration of antibiotics
   d. broad-spectrum antibiotics

2. Signs and symptoms of superinfection caused by *Candida* include:
   a. nausea
   b. sore mouth
   c. vaginal discharge
   d. all of the above

3. The recommended dosing schedule for amoxicillin is:
   a. every 12 hours
   b. every 4 hours
   c. every 6 hours
   d. every 8 hours

4. In debilitated patients, potassium depletion may occur with which one of the following:
   a. ampicillin
   b. ticarcillin
   c. pen VK
   d. cloxacillin

5. Impaired renal function can cause toxic accumulation of penicillins. Symptoms associated with decreased excretion include:
   a. ototoxicity
   b. pseudomembraneous colitis
   c. chills and fever
   d. seizures

6. Repository preparations of pen G should be given by:
   a. continuous intravenous infusion
   b. deep IM injection
   c. mouth
   d. intermittent intravenous infusion

7. The excretion of penicillins via the kidneys is inhibited by:
   a. allopurinol
   b. furosemide
   c. vitamin C
   d. probenicid

8. A serious adverse reaction that applies to all penicillin drugs is:
   a. ototoxicity
   b. anaphylactic reaction
   c. nephrotoxicity
   d. enamel hypoplasia

9. The prototype penicillin drug is:
   a. pen G
   b. pen V
   c. amoxicillin
   d. ampicillin

10. Penicillin antibiotics exert their antimicrobial action by:
    a. inhibiting protein synthesis
    b. inhibiting DNA synthesis
    c. inhibiting cell wall synthesis
    d. inhibiting cell membrane synthesis

11. The antibiotic that combines a penicillin derivative and a beta-lactamase inhibitor is:
    a. Bactrim
    b. Azo Gantanol
    c. Amoxil
    d. Augmentin

12. The penicillin most often prescribed for an acute uncomplicated urinary tract infection is:
    a. pen G
    b. cloxacillin
    c. ampicillin
    d. procaine pen G

13. The penicillin derivatives most effective in infections caused by penicillinase-producing organisms is:
    a. oxacillin
    b. cloxacillin

    c. dicloxacillin
    d. all of the above

14. The effectiveness of birth control tablets is diminished by:
    a. methicillin
    b. ampicillin
    c. ticarcillin
    d. carbenicillin

15. Compared to other penicillin derivatives, ampicillin causes a higher incidence of:
    a. nausea
    b. diarrhea
    c. photosensitivity
    d. nephrotoxicity

16. The percentage of the population thought to be allergic to penicillins is:
    a. 1 to 2%
    b. 3 to 5%
    c. 5 to 10%
    d. 10 to 15%

17–21. Matching:

Trade Name	Generic Name
17. _____ Amoxil	a. cloxacillin
18. _____ Bicillin	b. penicillin VK
19. _____ Polycillin	c. procaine penicillin G
20. _____ Tegopen	d. amoxicillin
21. _____ V-Cillin-K	e. ampicillin

CEPHALOSPORINS

22. Bleeding disorders have been associated with which one of the following cephalosporins:
    a. moxalactam
    b. cephalothin
    c. cephalexin
    d. cefaclor

23. A potential toxicity of all cephalosporins is:
    a. ototoxicity
    b. phototoxicity
    c. nephrotoxicity
    d. hepatoxicity

24. Which one of the following is available only as an oral preparation?
    a. Ancef
    b. Keflin
    c. Mandol
    d. Keflex

25. Patients receiving moxalactam should avoid:
    a. alcohol
    b. vitamin C
    c. milk products
    d. vitamin B_6

26. A patient, who is diabetic, is receiving Keflex for a urinary tract infection. Which one of the following urine tests will give a false positive for urine glucose:

a. Clinitest
b. Diastix
c. Testape
d. Ketodiastix

27. The third generation cephalosporins are considered to have a:
    a. broader spectrum of activity against gram-negative bacteria
    b. broader spectrum of activity against gram-positive bacteria
    c. higher incidence of anaphylactic reactions
    d. lower incidence of anaphylactic reactions

28. The cephalosporins are inactivated by enzymes, produced by resistant strains of bacteria, known as:
    a. microsomal enzymes
    b. transpeptidases
    c. polymerases
    d. beta-lactamases

29. Patients should be monitored for potential nephrotoxicity if cephalosporins are given with:
    a. Lasix
    b. probenicid
    c. clavulanic acid
    d. vitamin K

30. Allergic cross-reaction may occur in those individuals allergic to penicillins if given a cephalosporin. This statement is:
    a. true
    b. false

31–37. Matching: (Answers may be used more than once.)

Trade Name	**Generic Name**
31. _____ Ancef	a. cefonicid
32. _____ Keflex	b. cephalexin
33. _____ Anspor	c. cefazolin
34. _____ Kefzol	d. cephradine
35. _____ Velosef	e. cefamandol
36. _____ Mandol	
37. _____ Monocid	

TETRACYCLINES

38. In susceptible bacteria, tetracyclines:
    a. inhibit cell wall synthesis
    b. inhibit protein synthesis
    c. alter membrane permeability
    d. inhibit nucleic acid synthesis

39. Tetracycline is considered an agent of choice for:
    a. gonorrhea
    b. meningitis caused by *H. influenzae*
    c. Rocky Mountain spotted fever
    d. typhoid fever

40. The advantage of doxycycline over tetracycline HCl is:
    a. fewer adverse effects
    b. longer half-life
    c. better absorption
    d. broader spectrum of activity

41. It has been reported that approximately 50 percent of the patients who are prescribed minocycline will experience:
    a. dizziness
    b. blurred vision
    c. constipation
    d. dry mouth

42. A man is taking doxycycline as a precautionary measure for travelers' diarrhea. You should advise him to:
    a. avoid products that acidify the urine
    b. take the medication on an empty stomach
    c. avoid direct sunlight
    d. discontinue the drug and call the doctor if unexplained bleeding occurs

43. Prior to prescribing a tetracycline antibiotic, it is important to ascertain if the individual is:
    a. diabetic
    b. allergic to penicillin
    c. pregnant
    d. taking birth control tablets

44. An individual is taking Sumycin 250 mg qid for a sinus infection and is experiencing gastric upset. Should you advise the patient to take an antacid prior to each dose?
    a. yes
    b. no

AMINOGLYCOSIDES

45. The most serious side effects of aminoglycosides are:
    a. hypersensitivity reactions and ototoxicity
    b. ototoxicity and hepatotoxicity
    c. ototoxicity and nephrotoxicity
    d. nephrotoxicity and hypersensitivity reactions

46. Aminoglycosides are poorly absorbed from the GI tract; however, two are routinely given orally for bowel sterilization. They are:
    a. streptomycin and neomycin
    b. neomycin and kanamycin
    c. kanamycin and tobramycin
    d. tobramycin and amikacin

47. The aminoglycosides are principally used:
    a. to treat patients with hypersensitivity reactions to penicillins
    b. to treat tuberculosis
    c. to treat gram-negative infections
    d. to treat meningitis caused by gram-positive bacteria

48. Aminoglycosides should be used cautiously in patients who have:
    a. myasthenia gravis
    b. Parkinson's disease
    c. Addison's disease
    d. Crohn's disease

SULFONAMIDES AND TRIMETHOPRIM

49. Sulfasalazine is a rational choice in the treatment of chronic inflammatory bowel disease because of its:

a. increased systemic absorption
b. minimal systemic absorption
c. decreased incidence of GI upset
d. decreased incidence of skin rashes

50. Sulfisoxazole and sulfamethoxazole may be combined with phenazopyridine for its:
    a. synergistic effect
    b. potentiating effect
    c. analgesic effect
    d. none of the above

51–55. Matching: (Use each answer only once.)

Generic Name	Trade Name
51. _____ sulfamethoxazole	a. Azulfidine
52. _____ sulfacetamide sodium	b. Gantanol
	c. Sodium Sulamyd
53. _____ silver sulfadiazine	d. Silvadene
54. _____ sulfisoxazole	e. Gantrisin
55. _____ sulfasalazine	

URINARY TRACT ANTISEPTICS AND PHENAZOPYRIDINE

56. Prior to the initiation of drug therapy for a urinary tract infection, it is important for the nurse to:
    a. obtain a clean catch urine specimen for culture and sensitivity tests
    b. obtain an accurate drug history
    c. determine if the individual, if a woman, is pregnant
    d. all of the above

57. Which one of the following anti-infective agents used for urinary tract infections should be taken with food or milk to minimize GI upset and enhance systemic absorption?
    a. nitrofurantoin
    b. nalidixic acid
    c. trimethoprim
    d. methenamine mandelate

58. Methenamine mandelate is therapeutically more effective if the urine is maintained at a pH of:
    a. 5.5
    b. 7.5
    c. 9.5
    d. 10

59–62. Matching:

Drug	Mechanism of Action
59. _____ trimethoprim	a. mechanism not known
60. _____ nitrofurantoin	b. inhibits DNA synthesis
61. _____ metronidazole	c. prevents activation of folic acid
62. _____ methenamine	d. converted to formaldehyde

MISCELLANEOUS ANTI-INFECTIVE DRUGS

63. Although chloramphenicol is an excellent antibiotic with a broad spectrum of activity, it is usually held in reserve because of its toxicities. The toxic effect that is not reversible and usually fatal is:

  a. megaloblastic anemia
  b. leukopenia
  c. thrombocytopenia
  d. aplastic anemia

64. Erythromycin is considered the drug of choice for:
  a. Legionnaire's disease
  b. anaerobic central nervous system infections
  c. typhoid fever
  d. typhus

65. Erythromycin base is often given with neomycin for which of the following?
  a. encephalopathy caused by liver cirrhosis
  b. bowel sterilization prior to surgery
  c. gram-negative urinary tract infections
  d. severe otitis media

66. Which one of the following erythromycins has been associated with cholestatic hepatitis?
  a. erythromycin ethylsuccinate
  b. erythromycin estolate
  c. erythromycin gluceptate
  d. erythromycin stearate

67. A patient on your unit is being treated with clindamycin 150 mg PO q6h for an infection due to an anaerobic bacterium. You should discontinue the medication and notify the physician promptly if you observe:
  a. output less than input
  b. diarrhea with blood and mucus
  c. loss of deep tendon reflexes
  d. respiratory paralysis

68. A topical application of clindamycin for acne does not produce the serious side effects associated with oral administration.
  a. true
  b. false

69. Mr. A. is having dinner with some friends. He decides to have scotch and soda prior to the meal. After a few swallows he becomes flushed and nauseous and excuses himself because he is "not feeling well." Which one of the following would you associate with this reaction to alcohol?
  a. ampicillin
  b. cephalexin
  c. chloromycetin
  d. metronidazole

ANTIFUNGAL AGENTS

70. Amphotericin is administered intravenously for serious systemic fungal infections. One of the adverse effects associated with its use is:
  a. hepatotoxicity
  b. cardiotoxicity
  c. nephrotoxicity
  d. ototoxicity

71. Which one of the following antifungal drugs comes as a topical preparation, vaginal tablet, an oral suspension, and an oral tablet?
  a. flucytosine
  b. griseofulvin

    c. nystatin
    d. miconazole

72. A significant interaction that inhibits absorption occurs between ketoconazole and:
    a. cimetidine
    b. probenicid
    c. milk and milk products
    d. vitamin C

73. After amphotericin B is mixed for parenteral administration, the solution is:
    a. protected from light
    b. not refrigerated
    c. stored in a glass bottle
    d. administered immediately

ANTIVIRAL AGENTS

74. Solutions for IV infusion of vidarabine are not stored in the refrigerator prior to administration.
    a. true
    b. false

75. As an antiviral agent, amantadine can be used for the prevention of:
    a. herpes simplex
    b. varicella zoster
    c. influenza
    d. none of the above

76–79. Matching:

Antiviral Agent	Route of Administration
76. _____ vidarabine	a. PO only
77. _____ acyclovir	b. IV topically, and PO
78. _____ amantadine	c. ophthalmic ointment
79. _____ idoxuridine	d. ophthalmic ointment and IV

80–84. Matching: (Answers may be used more than once.)

Side or Adverse Effect	Drug
80. _____ gray syndrome	a. erythromycin
81. _____ enamel hypoplasia	b. ampicillin
82. _____ severe chills and fever	c. chloramphenicol
83. _____ irreversible bone marrow depression	d. amphotericin B
84. _____ drug of choice for *H. influenzae* meningitis (in addition to chloramphenicol)	e. tetracycline

=17=

Antineoplastic Agents

Since the introduction of the first antitumor agents in the 1940s, the use of chemotherapy in the management of cancer has evolved from one of last resort to an initial treatment of choice in many cases. The progress in chemotherapy can be attributed to better understanding of the disease itself, treatment regimens using more than one antineoplastic agent, and improvements in dosing and treatment scheduling.

A comprehensive discussion of neoplastic disease is well beyond the scope of this workbook. Suffice it to say, however, that neoplastic growth represents cells that have lost their response to the normal regulatory mechanism that signals them to stop growing. The neoplastic cells have undergone a genetic change of some unknown etiology, which renders them unresponsive to normal cell growth restraints.

Antineoplastic agents may be classified according to their mechanism of action or their origin. Agents are usually classified as alkylating agents, antimetabolites, natural products, and hormones and antihormonal agents. In addition, there is a miscellaneous category that is comprised of agents that do not fit in any of the classes listed. Agents may also be classed as cell cycle-specific or cell cycle-nonspecific agents. This means that some agents exert their cytotoxic effect only during certain phases of the cell cycle while others are cytotoxic throughout the cell cycle. A representation of the cell cycle is given in Figure 17–1.

In this chapter, the method of presentation will depart from the usual format used so far. The discussion will focus on the classes of agents rather than the individual agents. In order to avoid being repetitious, toxicities and nursing implications will be presented once after all the classes have been discussed. Use, specific precautions, and adverse effects are listed in Tables 17–1 through 17–5 for easy reference. A summary of the various mechanisms of action of these agents is shown in Figure 17–2.

For an excellent resource on this topic the reader is referred to *Cancer Chemotherapy, A Manual for Nurses,* by Teresa M. Berhen, published by Little, Brown and Company.

ALKYLATING AGENTS

Action and Fate. Alkylating agents interact with DNA in a way very similar to that of ionizing radiation. Their interaction may cause abnormal base pairing, cross-linking within the DNA molecule, or fragmentation of the DNA. Any one of these effects will result in incorrect DNA replication and incorrect RNA and protein synthesis causing cell death. The cytotoxic effect of the alkylating agents is not dependent on the cells being in a particular phase of the cell cycle. Most agents are metabolized in the liver. Mechlorethamine will spontaneously transform into metabolites once in solution.

Uses. For the uses of alkylating agents, please refer to Table 17–1.

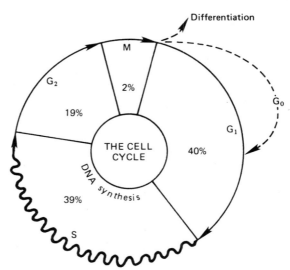

Figure 17–1. The cell cycle showing the various phases. *(From Meyers FH, Jawetz E, Goldfien A (eds): Review of Medical Pharmacology, 7th ed. Los Altos, Calif, Lange Medical Publications, 1980, with permission.)*

TABLE 17–1. ALKYLATING AGENTS

Generic Name	Trade Name	Route of Administration	Indications	Comments
Nitrogen mustards				
mechlorethamine (nitrogen mustard, HN_2)	Mustargen	IV push	Hodgkin's and non-Hodgkin's lymphomas; lung carcinomas	Avoid extravasation; administer within 15–30 min after mixing, administer over several minutes into a running IV; phlebitis and thrombosis common; amenorrhea and azoospermia common
chlorambucil	Leukeran	PO	Chronic lymphocytic leukemia; non-Hodgkin's lymphoma	Amenorrhea and azoospermia common
cyclophosphamide (CTX)	Cytoxan	IV, PO	Breast, lung, ovary, testis, bladder carcinomas; bone and soft tissue sarcomas; Hodgkin's and non-Hodgkin's lymphomas; acute and chronic lymphocytic leukemia; neuroblastoma and Wilm's tumor; multiple myeloma	Hemorrhagic cystitis may occur, frequency diminished with adequate hydration and voiding, administer drug early in the day; reversible alopecia common; amenorrhea and azoospermia common
melphalan	Alkeran	PO	Multiple myeloma; breast, ovary, testis carcinomas	Alopecia rare
Alkyl sulfonates				
busulfan	Myleran	PO	Chronic granulocytic leukemia	Ovarian suppression and amenorrhea common; weekly blood counts recommended while on therapy, discontinue if leukocyte count below 15,000
Ethylenimines				
thiotepa	Thio-Tepa	IM, IV, IT, intracavity, intravesically	Superficial papillary carcinoma of the bladder; malignant peritoneal or pleural effusions	Amenorrhea and azoospermia common

continued

TABLE 17–1. (*Cont.*)

Generic Name	Trade Name	Route of Administration	Indications	Comments
Triazene				
dacarbazine (DIC)	DTIC-Dome	IV, IA	Melanoma; all soft tissue sarcomas; Hodgkin's lymphoma	Patient may complain of pain or burning at infusion site, may be reduced by further dilution of solution or infusing at a slower rate
Nitrosoureas				
carmustine (BCNU)	BiCNU	IV	Lung, colorectal, stomach carcinomas; Hodgkin's and non-Hodgkin's lymphomas; brain tumors; multiple myeloma; melanoma	Skin contact with agent causes brown discoloration
lomustine (CCNU)	CeeNU	PO	Lung and kidney carcinomas; Hodgkin's and non-Hodgkin's lymphomas; melanoma	Take 1 hour before or 2 hours after meals to ensure adequate absorption

TABLE 17–2. ANTIMETABOLITES

Generic Name	Trade Name(s)	Route of Administration	Indications	Comments
Folic acid antagonist				
methotrexate (MTX)	Mexate	IV, IM PO, IT	Breast, head and neck, lung, gastrointestinal, gestational trophoblastic carcinomas; acute lymphocytic leukemia; meningeal leukemia; osteosarcoma[a] (high dose)	Use preservative-free diluent for IT and high dose dilution; antidote for high dose protocol is calcium leucovorin
Pyrimidine antagonists				
cytarabine (Ara-C)	Cytosar	IV, SC, IT	Acute lymphocytic leukemia	Use preservative-free diluent for IT dilution
floxuridine	FUDR	IA	Hepatic metastasis of gastrointestinal carcinoma	Dose reduced with decreased hepatic function; heparin added to IA infusion solution; gastrointestinal pain or other GI symptoms are indication to discontinue drug infusion
fluorouracil (5-FU)	Adrucil Efudex	IV, IA, topical cream	Breast, colorectal, stomach, pancreas, esophagus, liver, bladder carcinomas; basal cell carcinoma of the skin	For IA and IV infusion same as floxuridine. For topical use advise to avoid exposure to sun
Purine antagonist				
mercaptopurine (6-MP)	Purinethol	IV, PO	Acute lymphocytic and juvenile chronic granulocytic leukemia	Do not use with allopurinol, increases toxicity of 6-MP
thioguanine (6-TG)	6-Thioguanine	IV, PO	Acute nonlymphocytic leukemia	—

[a] Very high doses of methotrexate are used in experimental protocols for the treatment of certain tumors. The dose in this case ranges from 100 mg/m^2 to 10 Gm/m^2. After the methotrexate is administered, calcium leucovorin is given to the patient to protect or rescue the nonmalignant cells. Calcium leucovorin is given to the patient until the blood levels of methotrexate fall below the toxic level. Since a large number of cells are destroyed during this treatment, the patient is also treated prophylactically for hyperuricemia. This protocol should not be attempted by inexperienced personnel or in facilities not equipped to monitor methotrexate blood levels very closely.

TABLE 17–3. NATURAL PRODUCTS

Generic Name	Trade Name	Route of Adminis-tration	Indications	Comments
Vinca alkaloids				
vinblastine (VLB)	Velban	IV	Testicular, gestational trophoblastic carcinomas; Hodgkin's and non-Hodgkin's lymphomas	Avoid extravasation; monitor daily for neurotoxicity[a]
vincristine (VCR)	Oncovin	IV	Breast carcinoma; Hodgkin's and non-Hodgkin's lymphomas; acute lymphocytic leukemia; Wilms' tumor, neuroblastoma, rhabdomyosarcoma, Ewing's sarcoma; multiple myeloma	Avoid extravasation, low incidence of neurotoxicity; maximum weekly dose = 2 mg
Antibiotics				
bleomycin	Blenoxane	IV, IM, IA, SC	Testis, head and neck, penis, cervix, vulva, anus, skin, and lung carcinomas; Hodgkin's and non-Hodgkin's lymphomas	Watch for anaphylactic reaction, especially in lymphoma patients; assess pulmonary function frequently; life time culmulative dose = 400 units; reduce dose for renal failure
dactinomycin	Cosmegen	IV	Gestational trophoblastic and testis carcinomas; Wilms' tumor, rhabdomyosarcoma, Ewing's sarcoma	Avoid extravasation; alopecia common
daunorubicin	Cerubidine	IV	Acute nonlymphocytic leukemia	Avoid extravasation; cardiotoxic, monitor heart function; maximum life time dose = 550 mg/m^2; reduce dose for liver or kidney impairment; alopecia common; causes red discoloration of urine
doxorubicin	Adriamycin	IV	Breast, bladder, lung, prostate, stomach, and thyroid carcinomas; bone and soft tissue sarcomas; Hodgkin's and non-Hodgkin's lymphomas; acute lymphocytic and nonlymphocytic leukemias; Wilms' neuroblastoma and rhabdomyosarcoma	Avoid extravasation; cardiotoxic,[b] monitor heart function; maximum life time dose = 550 mg/m^2; reduce dose for liver impairment; alopecia common; causes red discoloration of urine
mithramycin	Plicamycin (formerly Mithracin)	IV	Testis carcinoma; severe refractory hypercalcemia	Avoid extravasation; infuse slowly to avoid GI toxicity; monitor for flushing, may signal impending bleeding crisis
mitomycin (mitomycin C)	Mutamycin	IV	Stomach and pancreas carcinomas	Avoid extravasation; alopecia common; solution stable 3 hr in D$_5$W and 12 hr in NS
Podophyllotoxin derivatives				
etoposide (VP-16)	VePesid	IV	Small oat lung carcinoma; nonlymphoblastic leukemia; testis carcinoma	Infuse over at least 30–60 min to avoid severe hypotension; monitor blood pressure frequently during infusion

[a] Signs of neurotoxicity include paresthesias of hands and feet, loss of deep tendon reflex, mental depression, ptosis, double vision, neuritic pain, motor difficulties. Monitor patient daily for muscular weakness in hands and loss of deep tendon reflexes. Depression of Achilles' tendon reflex early sign of neurotoxicity.

[b] Signs of cardiac toxicity include dyspnea, edema, hypotension, rapid pulse, arrhythmias. Cardiac function should be tested prior to initiation of treatment with either daunorubicin or doxorubicin, and monitored periodically during treatment.

TABLE 17–4. MISCELLANEOUS AGENTS

Generic Name	Trade Name	Route of Adminis-tration	Indications	Comments
asparaginase (L-asparaginase)	Elspar	IV, IM	Acute lymphocytic leuke-mia	Mild to severe hypersensi-tivity reactions, be prepared to treat anaphylaxis
cisplatin (CDDP)	Platinol	IV, IA	Testis, ovary, bladder, head and neck, and lung carcinomas	Irreversible nephrotoxicity may occur if patient not adequately hydrated; final solution should be in chloride-containing fluid, diuresis enhanced with furosemide or mannitol
hydroxyurea	Hydrea	PO	Head and neck carcino-mas; chronic granulo-cytic leukemia; acute lymphocytic and non-lymphocytic leukemia	Daily dose adjusted according to blood counts
procarbazine	Matulane	PO	Lung carcinoma; Hodgkin's and non-Hodgkin's lymphomas	Food and drug interac-tions possible: avoid ethanol, CNS depres-sants, sympathomi-metics, antidepressants, and tyramine-rich foods

TABLE 17–5. HORMONAL AND ANTIHORMONAL AGENTS

Generic Name	Trade Name(s)	Route of Adminis-tration	Indications	Comments
Adrenalcorticosteroids				
dexamethasone	Decadron Hexadrol	PO, IV	Cerebral edema	Suppression of adrenal function, must taper off medication; K^+ depletion, Na^+ reten-tion; edema; drug-induced Cushing's syndrome; increased risk of fungal and bacterial infections; euphoria, depression; epigastric pain, peptic ulcers
prednisone	Deltasone	PO, IV	Breast carcinoma; acute and chronic lympho-cytic leukemias; Hodgkin's and non-Hodgkin's lymphomas; multiple myeloma	Same as Decadron
Androgens				
fluoxymesterone	Halotestin	PO	Breast carcinoma	Hypercalcemia may occur initially; mascu-linization of females; mild fluid retention
testolactone and others	Teslac	PO	Same	Same
Estrogens				
chlorotrianisene	Tace	PO	Prostate carcinoma	Fluid retention and edema; hypercalce-mia initially; nausea and vomiting; Na^+ retention and edema; increased risk for thromboemboli; feminization in males
diethystilbestrol (DES)	—	PO	Breast and prostate carcinomas	Same

continued

TABLE 17–5. (Cont.)

Generic Name	Trade Name(s)	Route of Adminis-tration	Indications	Comments
diethylstilbestrol diphosphate	Stilphostrol	IV	Same	Same
Progestins				
hydroprogesterone caproate	Delalutin	IM	Breast and endometrial carcinomas	Menstrual irregularities; hypercalcemia initially
medroxyprogesterone	Depo-Provera Provera	IM PO	Same	Same
megestrol acetate	Megace	PO	Same	Same
Estrogen antagonist				
tamoxifen	Nolvadex	PO	Breast carcinoma	Nausea and vomiting initially; hot flashes

ANTIMETABOLITES

Action and Fate. The antimetabolites are compounds that are structurally similar to molecules needed for nucleic acid synthesis. These agents may exert one of two actions. Some of the agents may inhibit enzymes essential in the synthesis of nucleic acids, or the compounds themselves may be mistakenly incorporated into the nucleic acid producing incorrect base sequences. Either one of these actions affects cell growth and eventually causes cell death. Antimetabolites are most effective against actively growing cells and specifically during the synthetic (S)

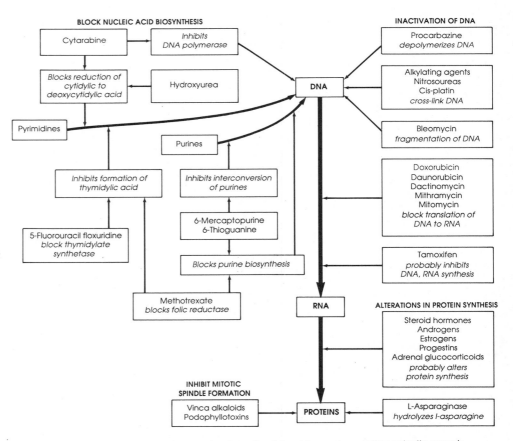

Figure 17–2. Summary of the mechanism of action of the various antineoplastic agents. (*Modified from Goldberg RS & Krakoff I: Hospital Formulary, Oct. 1979, p. 891, with permission.*)

phase of the cell's growth cycle (Fig. 17–2). All agents except methotrexate are metabolized in the liver before being excreted. Methotrexate is cleared by the kidneys.

Uses. For the uses of antimetabolites, please refer to Table 17–2.

NATURAL PRODUCTS

Vinca Alkaloids

Action and Fate. The vinca alkaloids are natural products derived from the periwinkle plant. They arrest cells at the mitotic phase of the cell growth cycle by inhibiting the formation of the mitotic spindle. For this reason these agents are most effective against actively dividing cells. Vinca alkaloids are metabolized by the liver prior to excretion.

Uses. For the uses of vinca alkaloids, please refer to Table 17–3.

Antibiotics

Action and Fate. This group of antitumor agents consists of agents that are the byproducts of various species of *Streptomyces,* a soil fungus. These agents affect the normal functioning and synthesis of nucleic acids. They can be cytotoxic during any phase of the cell cycle. Most of the antibiotics are metabolized in the liver prior to excretion. Dactinomycin is excreted unchanged. The exact means of excretion of bleomycin is not known.

Podophyllum Derivatives

Action and Fate. Etoposide is a semisynthetic podophyllum derivative obtained from the May apple plant. It arrests cell growth at the G_2 phase, which occurs just prior to mitosis (Fig. 17–2). Etoposide is cleared by both renal and nonrenal means.

HORMONES AND ANTIHORMONAL AGENTS

Action and Fate. The sex hormones (estrogens, progestins, and androgens) are useful in the palliative treatment of neoplastic tumors whose growth can be slowed because they have retained a sensitivity to hormonal control. Specifically the adrenalcorticosteroid, prednisone, exerts a direct cytotoxic effect against abnormal lymphoid cells. Tamoxifen is an estrogen receptor blocker, thereby blocking the effect of this hormone on tissue whose growth it stimulates.

Uses. For the uses of hormones and antihormonal agents, please refer to Table 17–4. (See Chapter 11 for the fate of these agents.)

MISCELLANEOUS AGENTS

Action and Fate. Since each of these agents exerts a different cytotoxic effect, the mechanism of action of each will be discussed individually.

Asparaginase is an enzyme that specifically destroys the amino acid asparagine. This action deprives leukemic cells of an essential amino acid and eventually starves them. Normal cells, unlike the leukemic cells, are able to synthesize asparagine and are spared.

Cisplatin has a mechanism of action similar to the alkylating agents. Hydroxyurea interferes with the final steps of DNA synthesis. The mechanism of action of procarbazine is not clear; it apparently has properties similar to the antimetabolites.

TABLE 17–6. VESICANT CHEMOTHERAPEUTIC AGENTS

Generic Name	Trade Name
dactinomycin	Actinomycin D
dacarbazine	DTIC
daunomycin	Cerubidine
doxorubicin	Adriamycin
mithramycin	Plicamycin
mitomycin C	Mutamycin
mechlorethamine	Nitrogen Mustard
vinblastine	Velban
vincristine	Oncovin

TOXICITIES

The toxicities that are most prevalent among the various antineoplastic agents are due to their ability not only to kill cancer cells but also normal dividing cells. Tissues in which growth is suppressed are bone marrow, the epithelial lining of the gastrointestinal tract, hair follicles, germ cell growth particularly in males, and fetal growth. Bone marrow depression is the major dose-limiting adverse reaction. The administration of most agents is associated with a high incidence of nausea and vomiting.

A less common adverse effect is a vesicant property that some of the agents have (Table 17–6). This property causes severe tissue necrosis if the agent infiltrates during infusion. Agents with this property are described as being extravasational.

Hyperuricemia is an indirect effect that may occur when an extremely large number of cells are killed. Precautions can be taken that lessen the consequences of this effect such as increased hydration, urine alkalinization, and administration of allopurinol.

Other toxicities that are agent specific are neurotoxicity (vinblastine, vincristine); hemorrhagic cystitis (cyclophosphamide); cardiotoxicity (daunorubicin, doxorubicin); pulmonary fibrosis (bleomycin); and anaphylactic allergic reaction (asparaginase and bleomycin).

NURSING IMPLICATIONS FOR ANTINEOPLASTIC AGENTS

The nursing implications that apply to the general aspects of chemotherapy are given first; the ones with more agent-specific applications are listed afterwards.

General Nursing Implications

Prior to the administration of any antineoplastic agent there are certain baseline data that should be obtained. These include vital signs, complete blood picture, electrolyte values, and specific organ function tests. In addition, the following should be monitored:

Bone Marrow Suppression

- Leukopenia

    Monitor vital signs.
    Assess patient daily for signs and symptoms of infection.
    Monitor blood counts.
    Minimize environmental risk of infection.
    Ask patient to report any signs of infection promptly.

- Thrombocytopenia

    Monitor vital signs.
    Avoid invasive procedures.

Do not administer IM injections.
Monitor platelet counts.
Avoid giving patient aspirin or aspirin-containing medications.
Instruct patient to avoid certain activities that may promote bleeding.

- Anemia

Monitor vital signs.
Monitor hematocrit and hemoglobin.
Patient may need increased rest periods.
Assess patient for shortness of breath, palpitations, and need for O_2.

Ulceration of Gastrointestinal Tract

- Examine the patient's mouth daily; assess for inflammation and white patches.
- Teach patient correct oral hygiene.
- Patient may require artificial saliva for xerostoma.
- For oral superinfection, patient may require local anesthetic to reduce pain (i.e., Viscous Xylocaine) or an anti-infective oral solution (i.e., nystatin).
- Patient should avoid spicy foods.
- Emesis and stools should be tested for occult blood.

Alopecia

- Counsel patient about hair loss.
- Assure patient hair will grow back, but may be of different texture or color.

Nausea and Vomiting

- Give antinauseants as directed.
- Try to schedule meals to avoid times of peak nausea.
- Help patient to maintain optimum nutrition.

Azoospermia and Amenorrhea

- Patient should be counseled about possible irreversible sterility.
- Male patient may want to learn about sperm banking.
- Advise patient to avoid conceiving during treatment.

Specific Nursing Implications

The following nursing implications are applicable to specific agents except the last implication referring to hyperuricemia. Hyperuricemia is a condition that occurs in certain chemotherapeutic protocols that use higher than usual doses causing a high cell mortality and thus a high blood level of uric acid.

Extravasation. (Refer to Table 17–6 for specific agents.)

- Ensure that line is patent before starting infusion.
- Monitor infusion site frequently.
- Assess infusion site for pain, burning, swelling.

Pulmonary Toxicity with Bleomycin

- Obtain baseline pulmonary function.
- Assess patient for dry cough, dyspnea, rales.
- Patient should not exceed a total life cumulative dose of 400 units.

Cardiotoxicity with Daunonubicin and Doxorubicin

- Obtain baseline cardiac function.
- Assess patient for clinical signs of congestive heart failure.
- For both daunorubicin and doxorubicin, the total life time cumulative dose should not exceed 550 mg/m².

Neurotoxicity with Vincristine and Less Commonly with Vinblastine

Assess patient for:

- Constipation, abdominal pain, paralytic ileus
- Jaw pain and hoarseness
- Weakness or numbness of arms, hands, legs, or feet
- Slapping gait
- Mental depression
- Assess daily for decreased or absence of deep tendon reflex
- Tinnitis

Anaphylactic Reaction with Asparaginase and Bleomycin

- Closely monitor patient during infusion of drug.
- Be prepared with appropriate emergency equipment and drugs in case patient does have a reaction.

Hyperuricemia

- Become familiar with precautionary measures which include increased fluid intake, alkalinization of urine, and the administration of allopurinol.
- Monitor serum and urine uric acid levels.
- Monitor and record urine pH.
- Assess patient for joint or flank pain, swelling of lower limbs and feet, and changes in input–output ratio.

Review Questions

1. The dose-limiting adverse reaction of the majority of chemotherapy agents is:
   a. bone marrow suppression
   b. gastrointestinal intolerance
   c. anorexia
   d. alopecia

2. As part of patient assessment, deep tendon reflexes should be checked daily when the patient is receiving:
   a. Ara-C
   b. Cytoxan
   c. Velban
   d. Adriamycin

3. After a course of high dose methotrexate, the patient is "rescued" from the toxic effects by administering:
   a. mannitol
   b. calcium leucovorin
   c. allopurinol
   d. sodium bicarbonate

4. During chemotherapy, large numbers of cells are often destroyed causing hyperuricemia. In order to facilitate the excretion of uric acid and avoid kidney damage, the urine pH is made:
   a. basic
   b. acidic
   c. not altered
   d. uric acid excretion is not dependent on pH

5. Drugs that are classified as extravasational agents are only administered:

a. IM
b. IV
c. ID
d. SQ

6. Azoospermia occurs most often with the majority of:
   a. vinca alkaloids
   b. antibiotics
   c. alkylating agents
   d. antimetabolites

7. Accidental skin contact with _____ will cause brown spots.
   a. BCNU
   b. Adriamycin
   c. 5-FU
   d. vincristine

8. Severe gastrointestinal symptoms are an early sign of toxicity and an indication to discontinue:
   a. procarbazine
   b. cisplatin
   c. Alkeran
   d. FUDR

9. A red discoloration of urine commonly occurs with:
   a. dacarbazine
   b. Adriamycin
   c. methotrexate
   d. dactinomycin

List four antineoplastic agents that can cause alopecia.

10. _____

11. _____

12. _____

13. _____

14. Anaphylactic reaction precautions should be taken with _____
    and _____ .

15. Ara-C should be diluted with preservative-free diluent when it is administered:
    a. IM
    b. SQ
    c. IV
    d. IT

16. To reduce nephrotoxicity, mannitol may be administered with which one of the following antineoplastic agents?
    a. Cytoxan
    b. thiotepa
    c. cisplatin
    d. bleomycin

17–25. Matching: Indicate whether or not the drugs listed in column A are extravasational.

Column A	Column B
17. ____Adriamycin	a. extravasational
18. ____cisplatin	b. not extravasational
19. ____Velban	

20. _____Oncovin
21. _____bleomycin
22. _____Cytoxan
23. _____mechlorethamine
24. _____Mutamycin
25. _____methotrexate

26–35. Matching: Please match the following drug names with the most applicable phrase in the second column.

Drug Name

26. _____Adriamycin

27. _____mercaptopurine
28. _____vincristine
29. _____mithramycin

30. _____cyclophosphamide

31. _____bleomycin

32. _____etoposide
33. _____procarbazine

34. _____Nolvadex
35. _____FUDR

Characteristic

a. patient must be well hydrated to avoid hemorrhagic cystitis
b. given intra-arterially only
c. dose should not exceed 2 mg/week
d. assess patient for rales and dry cough
e. flushing may indicate impending bleeding crisis
f. allopurinol enhances toxicity of this drug
g. dose-related hot flashes
h. monitor blood pressure during infusion
i. monitor cardiac function
j. avoid tyramine-containing foods

Appendix

COMMONLY USED MEDICAL ABBREVIATIONS

ac	before meals	MV	megavolts or millivolts
AD	right ear	ng	nanogram (1/1000 of a microgram)
ad lib	as desired		
AS	left ear	NPO	nothing by mouth
bid	twice a day	NVD	nausea, vomiting, diarrhea
BP	blood pressure		
bpm	beats per minute	NS	normal saline
c̄	with	OD	right eye
CBC	complete blood count	OS	left eye
CHF	congestive heart failure	p̄	after
CNS	central nervous system	pc	after meals
C&S	culture and sensitivity	PO	by mouth
CVP	central venous pressure	PRN	as needed
D/C or DC	discontinue	qd	every day
DOE	dyspnea on exertion	qh	every hour
D_5W	dextrose (5%) in water	q2h	every 2 hours
ECG	electrocardiogram	q4h	every 4 hours
GI	gastrointestinal	q6h	every 6 hours
Gm	gram	q12h	every 12 hours
hs	at bedtime	qid	four times a day
IA	intra-arterial	qod	every other day
ID	intradermal	qs	sufficient quantity to make
IM	intramuscular		
IT	intrathecal	Rx	prescription
IV	intravenous	s̄	without
IVH	intravenous hyperalimentation	SQ	subcutaneous
		SL	sublingual
IVP	intravenous push	SOB	short of breath
KVO	keep vein open	stat	immediately
L	liter	TO	telephone order
mcg or μg	microgram (1/1000 of a milligram)	TPN	total parenteral nutrition
		tid	three times a day
mEq	milliequivalent	VO	verbal order
mg	milligram (1/1000 of a gram)	VS	vital signs
ml	milliliter (1/1000 of a liter)		

Answers

Chapter 2

1. d
2. Antipsychotic agents block dopamine from interacting with its receptors in the brain; this results in similar symptoms found in Parkinson's disease. (See Chapter 6 for a discussion of Parkinson's disease.)
3. a. A condition in which the patient feels compelled to move about continuously.
   b. A group of symptoms characterized by facial grimacing.
   c. Stereotyped and involuntary movements characterized by sucking and smacking the lips, lateral jaw movements, and darting of the tongue.
4. b
5. a
6. b
7. a
8. a
9. a
10. a
11. b
12. a
13. b
14. b
15. a
16. b
17. c
18. d
19. i
20. a
21. l
22. f
23. b
24. j
25. c
26. d
27. g
28. h
29. e
30. k

Chapter 3

1. Reactive (secondary)
2. Endogenous (genetic)
3. Bipolar Effective Disorder (manic/depressive)
4. norepinephrine
5. serotonin
6. a

7. c

8. d

9–14. See Table 3–3 for answers.

15. b

16. Bipolar Effective Disorder (manic/depressive)

17. a

18–21. See Table 3–4 for answers.

22. g

23. i

24. h

25. b

26. c

27. f

28. d

29. e

30. a

Chapter 4

1. Less addicting

2. Greater margin of safety

3. Lack of effects on macrosomal enzyme activity

4. When used as hypnotics, they induce a more natural sleep, with more time spent in REM

5. a

6. d

7. a

8. e

9. c

10. d

11. d

12. d

13. c

14. c

15. b

16. a

17. b

18. c

19. a

20. a

21. d

22. d

Chapter 5

1. a

2. c

3. d

4. b

5. a

6. b

7. Increase the release of norepinephrine and dopamine from CNS neurons and block re-uptake of these neurotransmitters

8. Blocks re-uptake of epinephrine and norepinephrine

9. amphetamine complex, CII

10. benzedrine, CII

11. dexedrine, CII

12. (no trade name), CII

13. methylpheniclate, CII

14. benzphetamine, CIII

15. chlorphentermine, CIII

16. Tenuate or Tepanil, CIV

17. Preludin, CII

18. phentermine, CIV

Chapter 6

1.	c	14.	f
2.	d	15.	b
3.	c	16.	a
4.	a	17.	c
5.	Hallucinations	18.	e
6.	Confusion	19.	d
7.	Nightmares	20.	b
8.	Extrapyramidal movements	21.	a
9.	Tremor	22.	a
10.	Akinesia	23.	c
11.	Rigidity	24.	d
12.	e	25.	a
13.	d	26.	d

Chapter 7

1.	a,c	14.	d
2.	b	15.	c
3.	b	16.	Calcium gluconate
4.	b	17.	a
5.	b,e	18.	e
6.	a	19.	d
7.	c	20.	f
8.	d	21.	c
9.	a,e	22.	a
10.	a,c	23.	b
11.	c	24.	d
12.	b	25.	c
13.	b		

Chapter 8

1.	d	5.	c
2.	b	6.	d
3.	c	7.	c
4.	c	8.	e

9. f   15. j
10. d   16. k
11. i   17. g
12. a   18. b
13. l   19. c
14. h

Chapter 9

1. Brain   17. e
2. Spinal cord   18. c
3. Intestine   19. a
4. a   20. a
5. c   21. a
6. b   22. a
7. Respiration less than 12   23. e
8. Miosis of the eyes   24. e
9. Coma   25. c
10. c   26. b
11. b   27. b
12. a   28. b
13. a   29. a
14. a   30. a
15. a   31. Less gastrointestinal upset
16. c   32. Does not cause Reye's syndrome

Chapter 10

CARDIAC GLYCOSIDES

1. Digoxin has a shorter half-life, 36 hours, versus 5 to 7 days for digitoxin.

2. Digoxin does not require liver metabolism prior to excretion as does digitoxin.

3. c

4. Digitalizing a patient means that a loading dose of digoxin is calculated based on the patient's weight and kidney function. This dose is divided into 2 or 3 doses and administered in a 24-hour period usually every 8 hours. Blood levels of digoxin are determined between each dose in order to determine whether the therapeutic level has been reached. Administering digoxin initially in this way allows the health provider to achieve therapeutic levels of digoxin within 24 hours. Therapeutic blood levels would be reached in 5 to 7 days if digoxin is dosed once daily.

5. d

6. c

7. a

8. c

ANTIARRHYTHMIA AGENTS

9. b

10. c

11. a

12. c

13. a

14. d

15. a

16. e

17. d

18. g

19. f

20. a

21. b

22. c

23. h

ANTIANGINAL AGENTS

24. nitrates

25. beta blockers

26. calcium channel blockers

27. Nitrates relax all smooth muscle by direct action. This action is most prominent on vascular smooth muscle. The resulting vasodilation promotes the pooling of blood and produces lowered peripheral resistance, a fall in blood pressure, and a decrease in cardiac output. However, in the case of angina pectoris, the exact mechanism of action is not known, but it seems to be due to a reduction in the oxygen consumption of the myocardium.

28. d

29. c

30. d

31. b

32. c

33. d

34. Patients should be sitting or lying down when taking a sublingual tablet of nitroglycerin because the hypotensive effect of nitrates is intensified in the upright position.

35. Nitroglycerin tablets lose potency if stored in containers made of metal, plastic, or cardboard. Potency of the tablets is retained for a longer period of time if stored in a glass container.

36. Time and repeated exposure of nitroglycerin tablets to heat, air, and moisture will inactivate them.

ANTIHYPERTENSIVE AGENTS

37. ↑ 140/90 mm Hg, recorded at three separate times.

38. Kidneys

39. Heart

40. Brain

41. Eyes

42. acebutol (Sectral)

43. atenolol (Tenormin)

44. metoprolol (Lopressor)

45. b

46. e

47. c

48. a

49. d

50. f

51. g

52. d

53. a

54. a

55. d
56. a
57. a beta blocker
58. methyldopa
59. clonidine
60. prazosin
61. reserpine
62. hydralazine
63. captopril
64. guanethidine
65. minoxidil

DIURETICS

66. b
67. a
68. e
69. c
70. g
71. d
72. f
73. h
74. Site B
75. Sites A & B
76. Site C
77. Block sodium reabsorption
78. Block the action of aldosterone
79. Increase the osmolarity of the urine
80. Thiazide diuretics
81. Loop diuretics
82. Osmotic diuretics
83. Potassium-sparing diuretics
84. Carbonic anhydrase inhibitor
85. b
86. c
87. c

88. e
89. b
90. d
91. d
92. a
93. d
94. a
95. e
96. f
97. b
98. b
99. c
100. d
101. g
102. e
103. a
104. d
105. c
106. b
107. b

CALCIUM CHANNEL BLOCKERS

108. nifedipine
109. b
110. b
111. c
112. a
113. c

ANTICOAGULANTS

114. b
115. b
116. a
117. b

Chapter 11

1. b
2. b
3. c
4. c
5. d
6. a
7. a

8. b
9. a
10. b
11. b
12. c
13. a
14. d

Chapter 12

1. d
2. 72
3. a
4. c
5. c
6. b
7. a
8. a

9. c
10. d
11. c
12. a
13. b
14. d
15. d

Chapter 13

1. d
2. c
3. c
4. b
5. b
6. a
7. b
8. a
9. a
10. c

11. d
12. a
13. c
14. a
15. b
16. b
17. b
18. c
19. d
20. a

Chapter 14

1. d
2. c
3. a
4. e
5. a
6. c
7. d
8. b
9. a
10. d
11. alcohol
12. aspirin
13. indomethacin
14. methotrexate
15. phenylbutazone

Chapter 15

1. c
2. c
3. d
4. a
5. Pregnancy
6. Diarrhea caused by broad-spectrum antibiotics
7. Hepatic impairment
8. Nursing mothers
9. b
10. Overuse of laxatives leads to a dependence on these agents for regular bowel movements
11. Increase in exercise
12. Addition of fiber to diet
13. Increase fluid intake
14. d
15. d
16. a
17. b
18. c
19. a
20. b
21. a
22. b
23. e
24. e
25. e
26. e
27. b
28. c
29. c
30. b

Chapter 16

PENICILLINS

1. d
2. d
3. d
4. b
5. d
6. b
7. d
8. b

9. a

10. c

11. d

12. c

13. d

14. b

15. b

16. c

17. d

18. c

19. e

20. a

21. b

CEPHALOSPORINS

22. a

23. c

24. d

25. a

26. a

27. a

28. d

29. a

30. a

31. c

32. b

33. d

34. c

35. d

36. e

37. a

TETRACYCLINES

38. b

39. c

40. b

41. a

42. c

43. c

AMINOGLYCOSIDES

44. b

45. c

46. b

47. c

48. a

SULFONAMIDES AND TRIMETHOPRIM

49. b

50. c

51. b

52. c

53. d

54. e

URINARY TRACT ANTISEPTICS AND PHENAZOPYRIDINE

55. a

56. d

57. a

58. a

59. c

60. a

61. b

MISCELLANEOUS ANTI-INFECTIVE DRUGS

62. d

63. d

64. a

65. b

66. b

67. b

68. a

ANTIFUNGAL DRUGS

69. d

70. c

71. c

72. a

ANTIVIRAL DRUGS

73. a

74. a

75. c

76. b

77. d

78. a

79. c

80. c

81. e

82. d

83. c

84. b

Chapter 17

1. a

2. c

3. b

4. a

5. b

6. c

7. a

8. d

9. b

10. cyclophosphamide

11. dactinomycin

12. daunorubicin

13. doxorubicin, mitomycin

14. asparaginase, bleomycin

15. d

16. c

17. a

18. b

19. a

20. a

21. b

22. b

23. a

24. a

25. b

26. i

27. f

28. c

29. e

30. a

31. d

32. h

33. j

34. g

35. b

Glossary

Acetylcholine. The neurotransmitter of the parasympathetic and somatic nervous system.

Acidosis. A disturbance of the acid-base balance of the body with a shift toward the acid state.

Adrenergic. Refers to sympathetic neurons that release norepinephrine.

Adverse effect. An unintended, unpredictable, and potentially injurious response to drug action. Adverse effects generally result from direct toxic drug effects, idiosyncrasies, hypersensitivity reactions, and noncompliance.

Agonist. A drug with high affinity for the receptor and high intrinsic activity; causes a pharmacological effect by its interaction with a specific receptor.

Agranulocytosis. A decrease in or absence of agranulocytes (a type of white blood cell).

Allergy. An acquired sensitivity to drugs that involves an antigen-antibody reaction.

Alpha receptors. Adrenergic receptors that are stimulated by norepinephrine and epinephrine with the exception of the receptors of the heart.

Analgesia. Relief of pain.

Analgesic. A drug that lessens the sensation of pain.

Analgesic. A drug capable of relieving pain.

Anaphylactic reaction. A sudden, severe allergic reaction that causes hypotension, shock, bronchoconstriction, and often death, and constitutes a medical emergency.

Angina pectoris. Pain in the chest caused by myocardial ischemia. Usually occurs suddenly because of physical exertion or emotional stress.

Angioneurotic edema. Localized wheals or swellings occurring in subcutaneous tissue or mucous membrane probably as an allergic response to a drug or substance.

Anorexia. Loss of appetite.

Antagonist. A drug with high affinity for the receptor, but minimal or no intrinsic activity. Capable of preventing or reducing activity at the receptor sight. May also be called a blocking agent.

Antibacterial. Against bacteria.

Antibiotic. A drug that destroys or slows the multiplication rate of organisms.

Anticholinergic. A drug that antagonizes the interaction of acetylcholine with its receptor, resulting in a decrease of parasympathetic activity.

Anticoagulant. A drug that decreases the ability of the blood to clot or coagulate.

Anticonvulsant. Any drug that will stop a convulsion or epileptic seizure.

Antiemetic. A drug given to relieve or prevent nausea and vomiting.

Antiepileptic. Any drug that, when given prophylactically, will prevent or lessen the incidence of epileptic seizures.

Antimicrobial. A drug that prevents the multiplication of microorganisms.

Antineoplastic. Any substance or drug that prevents or inhibits the growth of cancerous cells or tumors.

Antipyretic. A drug capable of reducing an elevated body temperature (fever).

Aplastic anemia. A blood disorder caused by damage to the bone marrow resulting in a marked reduction in the number of red blood cells and some white cells.

Arterioles. Small arteries.

Ataxia. Muscular incoordination.

Bacteriocidal. Any antimicrobial drug that kills bacteria.

Bacteriostatic. Any antimicrobial that arrests or inhibits the growth of bacteria.

Beta receptors. Adrenergic receptors that produce inhibition or relaxation when stimulated by epinephrine (beta 2 receptors) and the adrenergic receptors of the heart (beta 1 receptors) that produce excitation when stimulated by epinephrine.

Bioavailability. The fraction of unchanged drug that reaches the systemic circulation.

Biotransformation. Metabolic changes that occur following drug absorption and distribution convert the drug into products that are usually less active and that can be more readily excreted.

Bradycardia. Slow pulse rate, usually less than 60 bpm.

Bronchospasm. Spasm or constriction of the bronchi resulting in difficulty in breathing.

Catecholamine. Generally refers to the neurotransmitters of the sympathetic nervous system, norepinephrine and epinephrine; also includes dopamine.

Carcinogen. A cancer-producing substance or drug.

Carcinoma. Cancer.

Chemotherapy. The use of drugs to treat infectious diseases and cancer.

Cholinergics. Neurons of the parasympathetic and somatic nervous systems which release acetylcholine.

Chronotropic. Usually refers to a change in heart rate, either positive (increased heart rate) or negative (decreased heart rate).

Cinchonism. A toxic condition characterized by headache, tinnitus, and deafness caused by overdose of cinchona alkaloids (quinine or quinidine).

Crystalluria. The presence of crystals in the urine, refers especially to crystals of the sulfonamide drugs, which cause kidney damage.

Diabetes mellitus. A disease condition characterized by a lack of insulin, which results in hyperglycemia, glycosuria, and ketoacidosis.

Diplopia. Double vision.

Diuresis. Production and passage of abnormally large amounts of urine.

Diuretic. An agent that promotes the excretion of water and electrolytes.

Drug metabolism. The biochemical breakdown of drugs in the body, usually in the liver.

Drug tolerance. A decrease in responsiveness to a drug after repeated or chronic administration.

Dyscrasia. A general term used to describe an abnormal condition of the blood.

Edema. The retention of excess fluid in body tissues.

Endogenous. Produced by the body.

Enzyme induction. Refers to the ability of some drugs to increase the amounts of metabolizing enzymes in the liver.

Epilepsy. A disorder of electrical activity of the brain resulting in the occurrence of periods of unconsciousness, seizures, and convulsions.

Epinephrine. Also referred to as adrenaline; it is the main hormone of the adrenal medulla that stimulates the sympathetic nervous system.

Exogenous. Originating outside of an organ or part; originating outside of the body.

Extrapyramidal symptoms (EPS). A group of symptoms consisting of pseudoparkinsonism (the slowing of volutional movements is also called akinesia: mask facies, rigidity, tremor at rest, and pill-rolling motions with the fingers); acute dystonia (abnormal posturing, grimacing, spastic torticollis, and oculogyric crisis); akathasia (compelling need to move without specific pattern, inability to sit still); and tardive dyskinesia (involuntary rhythmic bizarre movements of face, jaw, mouth, tongue, and sometimes extremities).

Extravasation. The escape of fluid into surrounding tissue causing damage to the tissue.

Fungicidal. Any substance or drug that kills fungi.

Fungistatic. Any substance or drug that inhibits the growth of fungi.

Glossitis. Inflammation of the tongue.

Glucocorticoids. Natural or synthetic steroid hormones (adrenal cortex) which alter glucose metabolism; these steroids are also used as anti-inflammatory drugs.

Glycosuria. The presence of sugar in the urine.

Grand mal. A serious type of epileptic seizure resulting in convulsions and a loss of consciousness.

Granulocytopenia. A reduction or decrease in the number of granulocytes (a type of white blood cell).

Half-life ($t_{1/2}$). The time required for drug concentration in plasma or total body to decline by one half. The concept of half-life is important in time determinations of steady state and clearance of drug from the body.

Hematuria. Blood in the urine.

Histamine. A substance found mainly in mast cells, which plays a vital role in mediating inflammatory and allergic reactions.

Hyperglycemia. An above normal increase in the blood glucose level.

Hyperkalemia. Above normal amounts of potassium in the blood.

Hyperlipidemia. An above normal increase in the lipid or fat level of the blood.

Hypernatremia. Above normal amounts of sodium in the blood.

Hypersensitive. Allergic.

Hypersensitivity reaction. An allergic reaction.

Hyperuricemia. Usually associated with gout in which there are abnormally high levels of uric acid in the blood.

Hypnotic. A drug that induces sleep.

Hypocalcemia. Below normal blood calcium levels.

Hypoglycemia. An abnormal decrease in the blood glucose level.

Hypokalemia. Below normal blood potassium level.

Hyponatremia. Below normal blood sodium level.

Hypotension, orthostatic. A decrease in blood pressure occurring after standing in one place for an extended period of time.

Hypotension, postural. A decrease in blood pressure following a sudden change in body position.

Idiosyncrasy. An unusual response to a drug caused by genetic variation.

Inotropic. Refers to a change in the force of myocardial contraction, either positive (increased force of contraction) or negative (decreased force of contraction).

Ketonuria. Ketones in the urine.

Leukopenia. A decrease in the number of white blood cells.

Lipoatrophy. Atrophy of subcutaneous fat caused by repeated injections of insulin in the same site, over prolonged periods.

Metastasize. The transfer or spread of cancer cells from one site (primary) to another (secondary).

Microsomal enzyme system. A catalytic system that generally inactivates drugs and makes them more water soluble so that they can be readily eliminated by the kidneys.

Mineralocorticoid. Refers to steroid hormones, like aldosterone, which regulate mineral (Na^+, K^+) metabolism and fluid balance.

Miosis. Pinpoint pupils; constriction of the pupils.

Myasthenia gravis. A disease of the neuromuscular junction resulting in muscular weakness.

Mydriasis. Dilatation of the pupil of the eye.

Myocardium. The muscle layer of the heart (adj., myocardial).

Necrosis. Death of tissue.

Neoplastic. New abnormal tissue growth, usually referring to malignant tumors.

Nephrotoxic. Harmful or damaging to the kidney.

Neurosis. A mental disorder involving an increased sense of fear and anxiety due to insecurity or some other psychological factor.

Norepinephrine. The neurotransmitter of the sympathetic nervous system.

Nystagmus. An involuntary and constant movement of the eyeball.

Oliguria. A decrease in urinary output.

Osteomalacia. A softening of the bones.

Osteoporosis. A loss of calcium from the bones, resulting in a decrease in bone density.

Ototoxic. An adverse effect of some drugs (diuretics, antibiotics) on the ear, resulting in deafness or vestibular disturbances.

Parenteral. Administration of a substance, such as a drug, by any route other than the oral route.

Paresthesia. An abnormal sensation such as numbness, tingling, or prickling, or heightened sensitivity.

Parkinsonism. A disease involving a deficiency of dopamine in the basal ganglia; symptoms usually include tremors, muscular rigidity, and ataxia.

Pharmacodynamics. Study of the time required for drug actions to occur in the body through processes of absorption, distribution, metabolism, and elimination.

Pharmacokinetics. The study of how a drug reaches its use of action and is removed from the body through processes of absorption, distribution, metabolism, and elimination.

Phlebitis. Inflammation of a vein.

Photophobia. An aversion to or intolerance of light.

Photosensitivity. Drug-induced skin changes resulting in unusual susceptibility to effects of sun or ultraviolet light.

Photosensitivity reaction. An exaggerated sunburn reaction when the skin is exposed to sunlight.

Physical dependence. The condition of being dependent on a drug (heroin or morphine), which when discontinued results in the abstinence syndrome.

Polydipsia. Excessive thirst.

Polyphagia. Eating large amounts of food.

Polyuria. Excessive production and voiding of urine.

Prophylaxis. Prevention.

Protein binding. A reversible drug-protein complex in equilibrium with free (active) drug in the plasma. Only the free drug can diffuse to the action site, thus factors that decrease protein binding (for example, displacement of bound drug by another drug, or hypoalbuminism) may raise the potential for increased pharmacological effect.

Pruritus. Itching.

Psychosis. A serious mental disorder involving a breakdown of personality and a loss of the sense of reality.

Salicylism. A toxic condition characterized by nausea, vomiting, and tinnitus caused by an overdose of salicylates (aspirin).

Sedative. A drug that reduces activity and produces relaxation.

Serum sickness. Symptoms of chills, fever, edema, joint and muscle pain, malaise.

Side effects. Effects produced by a drug that are in addition to the therapeutic effect.

Status epilepticus. A continuing series of grand mal seizures, which requires immediate medical treatment.

Stomatitis. Inflammation of the mouth.

Sublingual. Under the tongue.

Superinfection. A new infection caused by upsetting the balance of the body's natural flora.

Sympatholytic. A drug that inhibits or blocks the sympathetic nervous system.

Sympathomimetic. Acting like the sympathetic nervous system.

Synapse. The point at which the axon of one neuron communicates with the dendrites of another neuron.

Synthetic. Manufactured or produced by artificial methods, usually in a scientific laboratory.

Thrombocytopenia. A decrease in the number of platelets.

Thrombosis. Development of a thrombus.

Thrombus. A blood clot (pl., thrombi).

Tinnitus. Ringing in the ears.

Tolerance. Reduced responsiveness during repeated administration of a drug requiring increasingly larger doses.

Toxicity. Refers to the poisonous or toxic effects produced by drugs.

Uricosuric. Any agent or drug that increases the urinary excretion of uric acid.

Urticaria. Eruption of itching wheals, usually of systemic origin.

Vasodilation. Dilation of a vessel.

Vasopressor. A constriction of the blood vessels, which when widespread results in a rise in blood pressure.

Venous. Pertaining to the vein(s).

Venules. Small veins.

Vertigo. A sensation of moving or objects moving usually accompanied by difficulty in walking and maintaining balance.

Vestibular. Pertaining to the structures of the inner ear.

Bibliography

AMA Division of Drugs: AMA Drug Evaluations, 5th ed. New York, Wiley, 1983

APhA Staff: Handbook of Nonprescription Drugs, 7th ed. Washington, D.C., American Pharmaceutical Association, 1982

Becker TM: Cancer Chemotherapy—A Manual for Nurses. Boston, Little, Brown and Company, 1981

Billings DM, Stokes LG: Medical-Surgical Nursing, 2nd ed. St. Louis, C.V. Mosby, 1987

Billups NF, Billups SM: American Drug Index 1987, 31st ed. Philadelphia, Lippincott, 1987

Craig CR, Stitzel RE (eds): Modern Pharmacology, 2nd ed. Boston, Little, Brown and Company, 1986

Gillman AG, Goodman LS, Rall TW, Murad F (eds): Goodman and Gillman's The Pharmacological Basis of Therapeutics, 7th ed. New York, MacMillan, 1985

Guyton AC: Textbook of Medical Physiology, 6th ed. Philadelphia, Saunders, 1981

Hasten D: Drug Interactions, 5th ed. Philadelphia, Lea & Febriger, 1985

Kastrup ED (ed): Fact and Comparison. Philadelphia, Lippincott (Updated monthly)

Katcher BS, Young LY, Koda-Kimble MA (eds): Applied Therapeutics—The Clinical Use of Drugs, 3rd ed. Spokane, Wash., Applied Therapeutics, Inc., 1983

McEvoy GK, et al. (eds): American Hospital Formulary Service, Drug Information 86. Bethesda, American Society of Hospital Pharmacists, 1985 (Updated quarterly)

Physicians Desk Reference, 41st ed. Oradell, N.J., Medical Economics, 1987

Price SA, Wilson LM: Pathophysiology, 3rd ed. New York, McGraw-Hill, 1978

Thompson JM, McFarland GK, Hirsch JE, et al. (eds): Clinical Nursing. St. Louis, C.V. Mosby, 1986

Index